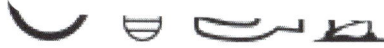

RA SEKHI

KEMETIC REIKI

Level Two

Ra Sekhi Arts Temple

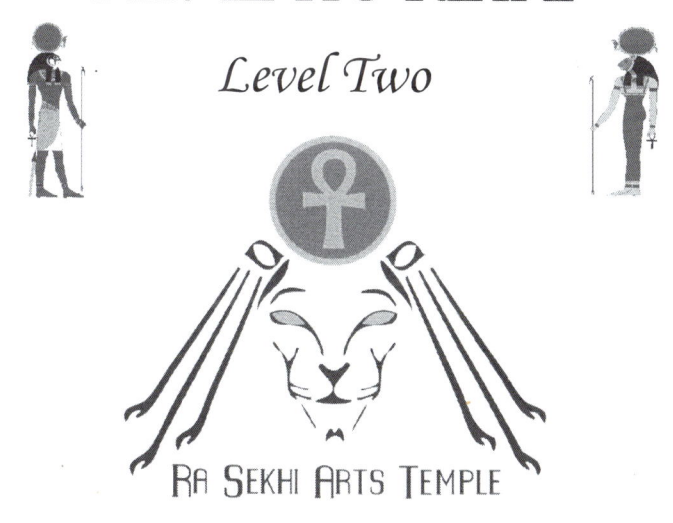

THIS IS A SACRED SYSTEM AND SHOULD BE GUARDED AS SUCH
ABOVE ALL TO YOUR OWN SELF BE TRUE
HONOR THE RA SEKHI SYSTEM
~REKHIT KAJARA ASSATA NEBTHET~
QUEEN MOTHER OF RA SEKHI ARTS TEMPLE OF HEALING

I dedicate this book to my first granddaughter Shamaya. May this work help to leave this world in a better place for you Beloved One.

Table of Contents

Preface	4
Energy Flow and Aurat	7
The Path of the Initiate	11
Sound Therapy	15
Hekau/Mantras	18
Crystals	21
Pendulums	28
Spiritual Protection	34
Altar Work	37
Ra Sekhi Symbols	39
Ra Sekhi Healing Session	47
Ra Sekhi Practitioner Hand Positions	52
Ra Sekhi Group Healing	56
Distance Healing	61
Procedures & Protocol	63
Hygiene & Appearance	67
Setting up your practice	68
Prayers	72
Testimonies	86

Preface

Now that you have done the work of healing yourself and cultivating your sekhem, it is time to move forward to sharing the healing energy with others.

Level 2 will give you more tools and the guidance to begin the work of healing others as a practitioner. You should now be familiar with energy and how it feels. You are aware of the aritu and the aura. You have been introduced to Sekhmet, your ancestors and Spirit Guides. The next lessons are meant to carry you to a higher level of energy healing. Level 2 is for those who have been helping people all their lives and want more tools to know how to help even more.

This books is a deeper step into energy healing. Each aspect we discuss could have a book written about them and we can not cover all of the information here. Your best teacher will be your experience working with the tools mentioned. Start with what stands out to you and begin your work there. This book is not meant to take the place of a class, but is a manual to work with after taking the class. You can feel the energy from the book, but it will not be as intense as it is when you are learning in the physical. Also the energy is traditionally passed from the teacher to the initiate in almost all forms of traditional healing all over the world. It was done this way for a reason. The interaction between the teacher and initiate is a divine relationship that allow the customs and order to be passed on and maintained as close to it's original form as possible. Some aspects of the work vary by individual, but there are some aspects that should be done a certain way every time. It is this and other nuances that make spiritual development and the teacher/initiate relationship important. Traditionally the initiate would honor and gift their teacher continuously for the lessons shared. The teacher or elder is representing the higher forces and maintaining the culture and knowledge of the ancestors. There is no price to equal the gift of spiritual awakening and enhancement. Yet we know there must be an energy exchange for all energy shared, whether on a conscious, subconscious, material or spiritual plane.

Do not allow fear to keep you from working with your healing gifts. Be confident and remember your were given these gifts for a divine reason. Some say that every family will have a healer. One who will remember and live by the ancient ways. The one they call the Black sheep. The one who remembers to work with the ancestors. The one who will seek truth and peace in life. The one who lives by and keeps the culture of the ancients. If you are reading this, that one is you. We thank you for coming forth to move forward in this way.

As melaninated people working with energy is innate, because our ancestors were so deeply connected to nature and lived with a higher consciousness. They mastered their energy and were able to project themselves, speak without words, move things with their minds, communicate with all of nature, etc....It is our right and our heritage to live in MAAT, with righteousness and balanced, positive energy. It is our duty to return to our natural Divine selves and restore MAAT within our lives and those with whom we are connected. I give thanks for this Divine Time and the Beautiful World which we are creating as we return to our Greatness and the Restoration of the Goddess on Earth.

THE POWER IS IN OUR HANDS!!!!!!!!!!!!!!!!

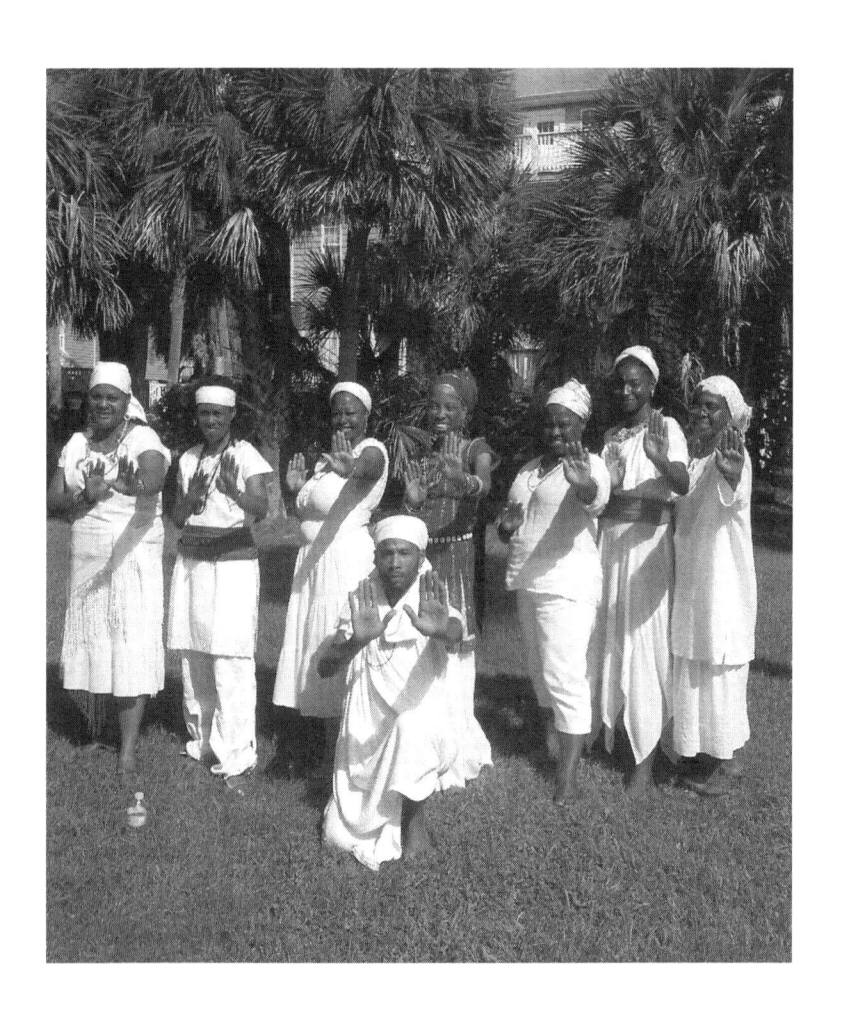

ENERGY AND THE AURAT

It is very important that we have an overstanding of energy in Ra Sekhi Healing. Energy is not created nor destroyed. It is in every living thing that was created by NTR. It is unseen but very real. It flows through our bodies like blood flows and it connects us with all of Nature. It is the vital force that gives us power to move, think and live. If we eat healthy, rest well and exercise we have strong energy, but our energy becomes weak if we don't live right. When we are happy, at peace and spiritually connected our energy is strong. When we are upset, stressed, depressed, angry, fearful, etc... our energy becomes weak.

We must be conscious of our physical, emotional, mental and spiritual energy. We must be able to master and manipulate our energy as our ancient ancestors did. Energy is effected by our senses; Sight, Taste, Balance, Hearing, Smell, Touch/Feeling, Time.

When we do energy work on ourselves. We use our personal energy, the energy of the Universe, the Spirit Guides, and the elements. (air, fire, water and earth). When we work on others we don't want to use our personal sekhem in this work. Our sekhem must be strong and balanced, but we must remain clear enough to allow the universal energy to flow thru us. Otherwise we may feel drained or feel the symptoms of our clients. A practitioner must know how to connect with higher forces to do the work.

It is important to work with all elements to generate wholistic healing of an individual. So during a healing session you want to use air using deep breathing or fire breaths. You can also sweeten the air with herbs/ incense to shift the energy. You also want to have a candle burning during the session to represent fire. Using holy water, florida water, spiritual baths, river water, etc or essential oils will represent air. Having crystals and plants around will generate the elements of earth.

You will also want to use these forces spiritually by invoking deities associated with the elements. Take time to learn about and how to work with other energies including Neteru, Orishas, Lwa, Loa, Nkisi as well as saints, guardian angels, elevated ancestors, etc. There is a universe of forces to work with in our healing practice. All of the Gods and Goddesses of Afrika are available to us as well as those of the Native Ancestors of North and South America. Start with your personal Ancestors and let them guide you. Remember as a Ra Sekhi healer we do not do work against another's will and we do not do work to bring harm to others. This energy will only work for the highest good of these involved.

We have an energy force field around our bodies, sometimes called the aura, which must be cleansed and kept strong with focus, prayer, chants, healthy lifestyle, etc. Our vital life force energy, Sekhem, flows through us through our Aritu, meridians and the Aurat sometimes called kundalini. In Kemet the Aurat is represented by two serpents (Uatchat-Nekhbet) in winding motion. They symbolize the electromagnetic waves that rise up on the left and right hemispheres of the brain reaching the pineal and pituitary areas. When we are able to raise our energy and aurat within we are rewarded with unlimited psychic-clairvoyant (spiritual) powers.

Nekhbet is the chief deity of upper Kemet. She is depicted as a woman wearing the White Crown and holding a lotus scepter intertwined by snake. She regulates the right side of the body, metalloids, acid PH, sunlight and heat.

Uatchat is the chief deity of lower Kemet. She is depicted as a woman wearing a red crown and holding a papyri scepter intertwined by a snake. She regulates the left side of the body, alkaline PH, moonlight and metals. The red fire is balanced with the white cooling energy. Therefore when the energy within us is flowing in harmony, we are balanced, at peace and are connected to all things natural.

When our Aurat is in harmony we can transcend all time and space and tap into the collective consciousness of the

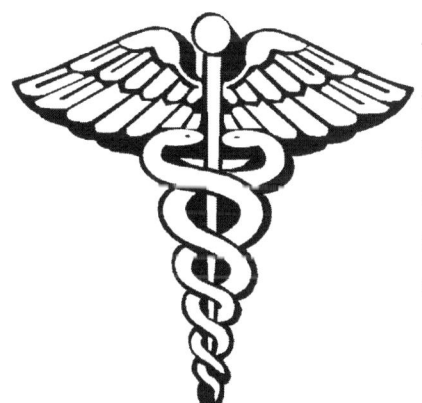

The symbol for the Aurat is used by the medical association today. It is an Ancient Kemetic symbol for wellness, oneness, higher consciousness, and balance of the lower and higher self. The wings represent ascension.

Ancient Ones. It is through focus, concentration, and practice that we are able to master, manipulate, and project our energy and use it to bring healing and balance in others. The Aurat is the symbol for the duality and the polar opposites that exists in all things. Our goal is to have complete balance within. We must find balance between our masculine/ feminine sides, left/ right, upper/ lower, light/dark, good/ evil, open/closed, sun/moon, etc.

We must also be conscious of the Hara Line which is known as the line that connects us with the ethers above our head and the energy of the earth below. It is a cord that runs through us along our spine. When we are conscious of this line, this connection we are able to connect with the universal energy, the ashakic records or the source of infinite wisdom and knowledge. It is through the hara line that we are able to project our energy to others and through time and space.

We also have energy meridians which flow through us and connect our organs to pressure points on our bodies. We can use these points to direct and balance our energy as well as others.

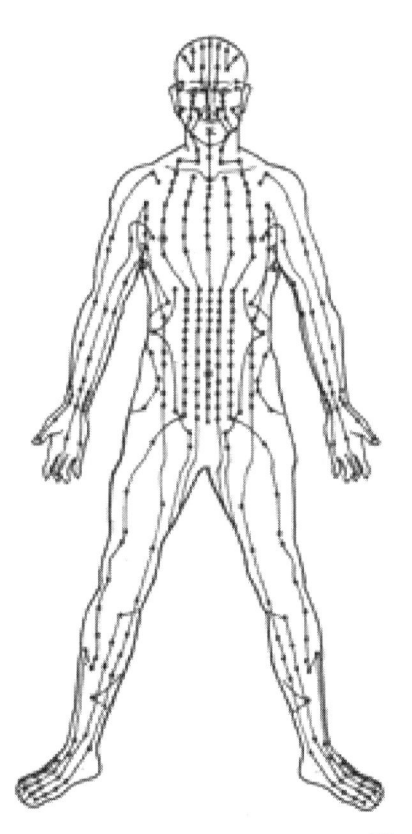

Acupressure point and meridian chart

THE PATH OF THE INITIATE

RA SEKHI practitioners use many tools to bring balance to our clients. The most important tool is the practitioner, their spirit and mind should be light, pure and positive. Other important tools are hekau (also called mantras), crystals, pendulums, symbols, sounds and the power to concentrate and focus.

One of the primary requirements of the spiritual aspirant is to be open-minded and humble enough to listen to the teaching of their Spirit Guides and teachers. THE 42 LAWS OF MAAT should be followed in order to purify the personality of egoism, anger, greed, lust, arrogance, and conceit, vanity, and pride. Following are the TEN VIRTUES OF THE INITIATE, which assist in the purifying process as well.

1. **Control your thoughts** Each of us have the opportunity to control our minds. We must know that all things in creation first begin with a thought. Then the words are spoken. Then the thought becomes manifest on the physical realm. We should be mindful of this truth and begin to change our way of thinking and speaking. Do not feed into negative thoughts and fears. You will attract what you are, your thoughts and feelings work like a magnet and will bring whatever you put energy into directly to you. It is a law of the universe.

2. **Control your actions** We have habits that may not be in alignment with our higher selves. When we become aware of truth we must act accordingly. For example if we say we are living in MAAT, we cannot continue to lie to our children about Santa Claus. We are responsi-

sible for what we know. The universe will hold us accountable in one way or another. We have to do better when we know better, even if it means doing things different from what we are used to.

3. **Have devotion of purpose** We all have a divine purpose for coming to the planet at this time. When you know what your purpose is you must work towards that everyday. Your job is not the work that you do to take care of yourself. Your job is to do the work that you agreed to do when you decided to come here at this time. If you don't know your purpose, ask your Spirit Guides to tell you. When you know your purpose you have to be dedicated to the mission. Work towards it everyday or as often as possible. If your work is a healer you have to help people and use the gifts you were given. Otherwise you may experience more challenges and obstacles on your journey. Your spirit guides will work to get your attention and help you to get on the right path.

4. **Have faith in your Spirit Guides ability to lead you along the path of truth** When you begin to pour libation and connect with your Spirit guides, you must know that they are working with you to assist you on your journey. When you get messages from the other side listen and follow with action. If you are unsure about the message you can always ask if this message is coming from The Most High. Have faith that your words, your prayers and your thoughts are heard and answered in the Universe.

5. **Have faith in your own ability to accept the truth** You must have faith and confidence in yourself as a healer. You know something is true when it is in agreement with your head and your heart. There are times when we must forget everything we learned in order to learn the truth. That doesn't mean that the lessons were wrong, it means that they served you for the time they were supposed to. On the path of ascension there is always more to learn, so you must be open to learn and accept even more.

6. **Have faith in your own ability to act with wisdom** To act with wisdom means to make choices based on research, intuition, advice from elders or oracle. It does not mean to act out of emotion or feelings. Think about your priorities and your goals when making decisions. Take you time and make choices that are for your highest good.. Following your intuition means following means following your first mind. Usually that is the voice of your higher self or spirit guides stepping in to assist you. Be confident that you are able to make good decisions.

7. **Be free from resentment under the experience of persecution (bear insult)** We know that people who are hurt will hurt others. As a healer we should not feed another ones pain with negative words or actions. That does not mean stand there and be insulted, it means be creative in finding ways to deal with someone who is rude or hurtful. Perhaps offer them a

healing session. Don't let their negative energy hurt or affect you. Recognize what is going on and stay at peace.

8. **Be free from resentment under the experience of wrong (bear injury)** We live in a violent world and many people do not know how to process their anger. As healers we must remember to be humble and nonviolent. Only in situations where we must defend ourselves or loved ones is it permissible to use violence against someone. Again we must find more intelligent and creative ways to handle our conflicts.

9. **Learn to distinguish between right and wrong** In this society it is hard to discern between right and wrong sometimes. However we must remember that we live according to the laws of MAAT which are very clear about what is right and what is wrong. Do good, choose righteousness.

10. **Learn to distinguish the real from the unreal** Most things that are real are things that we cannot see or touch. Love, Spirit, peace, harmony, joy. We live in world of illusions collecting stuff all of our lives, but we can't take any of it with us. Many people spend much money and energy on things that are not real. That is not in alignment with the path of the initiate. Do not be fooled by the illusions of this society.

To be initiated means to go from one level of consciousness to a higher level of consciousness. The process is life changing. You cannot be the best healer you can be if you are living and doing the things that everyone else is doing. Nor can you expect to do the same things you once did before your initiation. Working with energy is a serious thing. Commitment and dedication to your work and to your continuous healing is necessary. This is a chosen path for those who are meant to work with the spirit realm and continue the traditions of wholistic Afrikan healing. You should begin the process of help those around you first those in your immediate environment before working with others. This will build your strength and Ashe (spiritual power). It will also help keep the vibration in your home high which will also contribute to your success and your practice.

Sound Therapy

Sounds have a profound effect on our energy fields. Every tone we hear vibrates at a certain frequency which can effect us in positive or negative ways. In fact everything we hear whether from TV, radio or someone talking not only goes into our mind for us to process, but the sounds also affect our emotions, our spirits and our bodies as well. Each aritu/chakra is associated and responds to a particular tone. Some sounds are known to incite fear like the music we hear in a horror movie. Some sounds can bring peace like the sounds of nature or water running. Some music you listen to can make you laugh or cry, it's not just the words, it's also the energy patterns created by the sounds that shift our energy.

cry, it's not just the words, it's also the energy patterns created by the sounds that shift our energy.

There are many instruments that can be used for healing, including our voices. We use sound therapy to clear the aura and to balance the aritu. Instruments made in Afrika (drums, bells and rattles) work well with healing our people. Tuning forks and singing bowls are also powerful healing tools. Sounds that have more bass are grounding and good for balancing the lower aritu. Bells and sounds with a higher pitch work well with the higher aritu. It is good to let Spirit Guide you to know what sound will work better for an individual. You can also determine from the state of the aritu which sounds are needed to bring balance in a particular area.

Drums were used in Afrika to carry messages, to call spirits during ceremony, to call people and to heal. They assist one in reconnecting with the ancestors and with the true self. Drums can calm and soothe the spirit. They can also be stimulating, depending on the rhythm. Drums can also put one in a trance and can encourage astral travel as well.

Bells and rattles of all kinds can are good to remove blockages, to stimulate and activate the aritu, to restore balance in the mind and to dissipate negative energy. Bells are especially helpful to awaken one to higher consciousness and to call high spiritual forces.

Metal tuning forks, crystal and metal singing bowls are made to activate and balance specific aritu. Some instruments that we use in our practice are on the following page.

Instruments

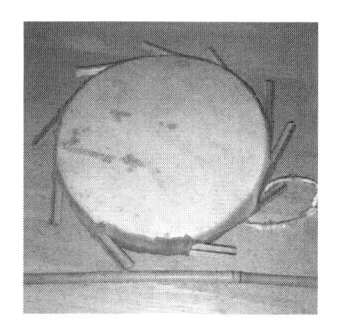

DRUM

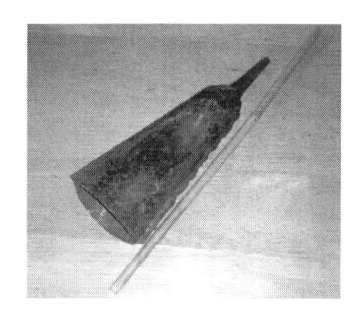

COWBELL

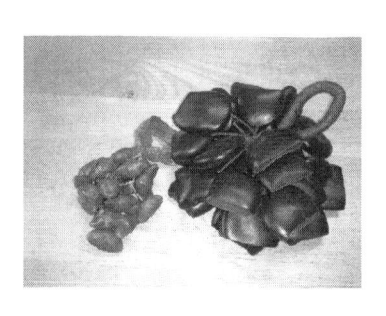

RATTLES

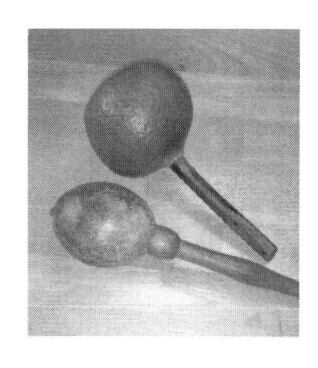

SHAKER

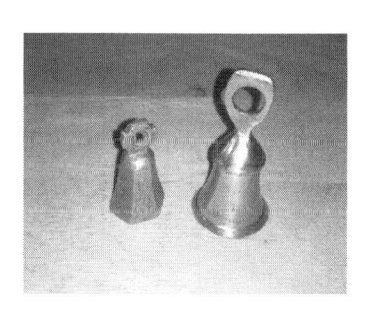

BELLS

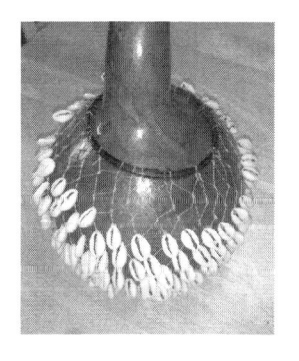

SHEKERE

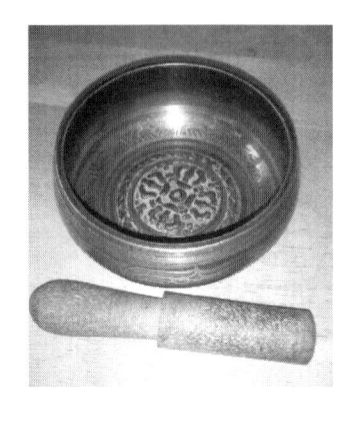

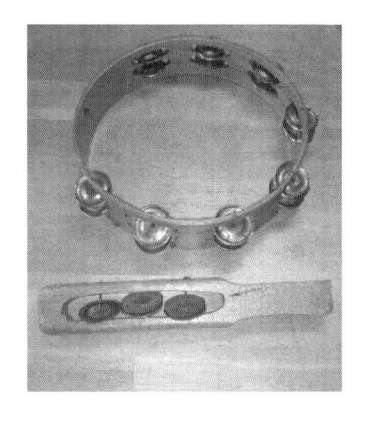

SINGING BOWL   TAMBORINE

Hekau/ Mantras

Hekau are words of power which are traditionally chanted repeatedly to increase and alter energy. All names for The Most High, Deities, Orisha, Ntru, and the symbols can be used as hekau. You can chant one or more of the names together to create a powerful song. Our ancestors would chant the same thing for an hour or more, or until they felt a change in the energy. Your pitch and rhythm are also important and will effect the vibration you put out.

Affirmations are words of power as well. We use the power of our voices and our words in our healing work to balance ourselves and clients in different ways. Make sure you say the affirmations with conviction. The energy you put into it will determine what energy comes from it. It is the frequency and tone of the sounds we make that bring forth changes in ones energy field and aritu.

The following list includes some powerful hekau and some of their properties

AMEN	calming, relaxing, elevating
RA	stimulating, activating, expanding
PTAH	strengthening, enlightening, creative
NTR	Divine/ sacred purification
KHM	grounding, cleanses, kidneys and liver
KHMRA	strengthens immune system
ASR	protective, resurrection, rebirth
AST	nurturing, soothing, cleansing
ANKH	life eternal and purity
SENEB	good health
HERU	action, willpower
SEKHEM	increases vitality
HETEP	invokes peace
MER	promotes unconditional love
SHAKTI	to dissipate negative energy

Also humming sounds such as zzzzzzzzzzz, oooooh-hhhhhh, mmmmmmmmmmm, ooooooo, aaaaaaaaaaa, eeeeeeeeeee, etc can be healing and balancing as well

Positive Affirmations are helpful for keeping your energy positive and strong. They can help to reprogram your mind. They can also be helpful to create things as we want them to be. Use them everyday or when needed. They can be used while working on clients as well to help them affirm their healing. You can use this example and create your own as well.

POSITIVE AFFIRMATION FOR MANIFESTATION

I HAVE RELEASED ALL FEAR, ANGER, AND GUILT FROM MY CONSCIOUS AND SUBCONSCIOUS MIND.

I HAVE SURRENDERED TO MY HIGHER SELF AND TO CHANGES WITHOUT RESISTANCE.

I HAVE ACCEPTED ABUNDANCE INTO MY LIFE WITH GRATITUDE.

I AM NOW A MAGNET FOR GOOD AND POSITIVE THOUGHTS.

I AM NOW A MAGNET FOR GOOD AND POSITIVE FEELINGS

I AM NOW A MAGNET FOR GOOD AND POSITIVE ACTIONS

ALL THAT I WISH TO MANIFEST IS MINE

I AM NOW IN A STATE OF RECEIVERSHIP FOR THIS

SO BE IT

Author unknown

MORE AFFIRMATIONS

I ATTRACT EVERYTHING THAT IS FOR MY HIGHEST GOOD

I AM HEALTHY, HAPPY AND WHOLE

I AM MORE HEALTHY EVERYDAY

I HAVE THE POWER TO HEAL MYSELF

I AM ONE WITH THE INFINITE SOURCE

I AM GUIDED BY DIVINE LOVE AND LIGHT

I AM FULL OF PEACE AND JOY

WORKING WITH CRYSTALS

There is a world of healing crystals available to use in RA SEKHI healing. They are very powerful healing tools. They have been used since ancient times, all over the world. They magnify the energy of the one wearing them as well as the environment they are in. The electromagnetic vibrations of each crystal are based on the minerals they are made of. They are very helpful in clearing the aura, balancing the chakras, balancing emotions, enhancing spiritual connection, protection against negative energy, astral travel, meditation and many more things. They are formed over hundreds or thousands of years so they also carry memory of past times. When working with crystals it is best to touch them or allow them to touch your skin. When you perspire while holding a crystal you are able to absorb the energy from the crystal even more. They are said to have healing qualities for the mind, body and spirit. Even if you wear a crystal and it doesn't touch your skin, you can still feel the benefits of its energy. They are also said to be even more powerful for melaninated ones, our melanin allows us to absorb and use the energy of crystals on a higher level than others.

Quartz is one that everyone should have at least one of. Clear quartz is known to radiate positive energy, it helps keep you clear, and it balances and activates the chakras. It is healing, activating, can raise your vibration and enhance your spiritual powers. It can be worn every day or in the home or office. It can transmute negative energy, so it should be cleaned often. There are many varieties of clear quartz, elestial quartz helps one connect with their highest self. Lemurian and Tibetan quartz are other varieties worth checking into, they are both said to be highly spiritual, highly charged and very powerful.

Another powerful and popular stone is amethyst. It can range from a deep purple to a light violet color and even clear or white. The color of the stone helps one determine the vibration of the stone. The stronger or darker the color the shorter the waves are so it moves quicker and feels stronger than more pastel like shade. Amethyst is known as an all heal crystal. It works with all chakras, but especially the crown. It can enhance ones spiritual connection and powers, so it is good to hold while praying or meditating. Sleeping with amethyst will enhance your dream state and wearing amethyst will protect you from negative influences and drama.

Citrine is another excellent stone to work with and to have around. It works to activate and stimulate your life force energy. It can clear your aura, your thoughts and emotions. It also transmutes negative energy. It is good to transmute negative effects of radioactive energy. Citrine is a powerful addition to crystal grids and can be used to clean energy from other crystals.

Because many crystals absorb energy it is important to clean them often, like once a month or every season if you work with them often. You can use natural things to clean crystals like sunlight, moonlight, seawater or rainwater, salt, lemon or berry juice can be used as well. You can also bury them in the earth and let them sit for 3 or more days.

Hard crystals like quartz can be clean with almost everything. Softer crystals like malachite, angelite, jade, infinite, selenite, etc....do not like to be cleaned with salt water, it will alter the color, texture and energy of your stone.

Black stones are important to have because they are the most powerful stones for absorbing negative energy, protecting against psychic attack and they are very grounding. You can choose between black tourmaline, which also protects against radiation, obsidian, jet or black jasper. Be careful with hematite which will sometimes break after absorbing negative energy or it may irritate your energy field and give you headaches (in some cases). Black stones are good to wear or keep in your home or office, to keep positive energy flowing in your environment.

Lapis lazuli is another good stone that has been used since ancient times. It can work to enhance your intuition and your ability to see clearly. It is soothing to the mental and emotions. It stimulates spiritual powers, protects against psychic attack, promotes harmony and stimulates your mind. You can place it on your first eye or throat chakra while meditating. Ask to see and speak more clearly or affirm that your psychic powers are strong. This is another good stone to sleep with to enhance your dream work.

Rose quartz is very good for working with the heart and issues of heart. It radiates unconditional love, self-love, harmony and peace. It is good to work with to balance and heal the heart and relationships. Many Sisters develop breast cancer because of heart/relationship issues that have not been processed properly. The heart becomes hard because of bitterness, sadness or anger; these emotions can lead to the development of tumors. Using crystals and other natural things to process that energy, thoughts and emotions can prevent those kinds of diseases. You can use rose quartz by holding it in your hand or putting it directly on your heart. Say affirmations of love, healing and forgiveness. Release negative thoughts and emotions and do this whenever you are feeling sad or angry to help change your vibration quickly.

There are other purple stones that are very good to work with charoite, sugalite and lepidolite. They all work with the crown chakra, they enhance your spiritual connection, promote self -love and assist you with connecting to your higher self.

There is another purple stone from South Africa called the spiritual mystic quartz it is also called a cactus quartz. It is made with amethyst, citrine and quartz and is super powerful. The colors vary but it is recognized by the crystalized patterns that surround the stone. It looks like hundreds of tiny crystals together to form a larger crystal, so each one is made of tiny universes that are connected. This stone is said to be very good to heal divisions within self, in families and communities. It is very good to use during healing sessions and especially with groups.

When I became aware of how crystals work, I placed them all around my home. I begin to notice that when people came to my house they would always say the home was peaceful, calming and welcoming. People seemed so glad to come and did not want to leave because the energy in the house was so positive. I attribute the peaceful vibe to the crystals and aromatherapy that I was doing at the time.

It is good to set up a crystal grid around your client before a healing session. This will allow the protective energy to remain in the healing space and magnify the healing session. Crystal Grids are made in certain shapes ; circle, square, diamond and can have one or more layers. Large stones work best. Protective stones like tourmaline, clear quartz, amethyst and citrine are good to use. You can create a love grid with rose and clear quartz. You can also make a crystal grid directly on your client for your healing session. Using more than one crystal at a time magnifies the energy and will add power to your healing work.

You want to program your crystals to work with you the way you need them too. After you clean them and hold them and talk into them. Share your needs and speak your intentions into them, ask them to work with you and share their healing medicine with you. There are many books about crystals but the best teacher is experience.

Follow is a chart with more crystal info

CRYSTAL	USED FOR	ARITU/CHAKRA
Tiger Eye	Protection, enhances psychic ability	Root, solar plexus
Mookite	Balances emotions, purifies blood	Root, sacral, solar plexus
Unakite	Promotes vision, enhances personal power	Heart, first eye
Labradorite	Raises consciousness, stimulate intuition	First eye, crown
Bloodstone	Purifies blood, banish negative, calming	Solar plexus, heart
Aventurine (green)	Promotes prosperity, compassion	heart
Jasper	Balances emotions	root
Topaz	Heals, stimulates, recharging	Sacral, solar plexus
Magnetite	Attracts, grounding	root
Turquoise	Protective, healing, raises spiritual energy	Throat, first eye

Carnelian	Grounding, stimulates creativity	Root, sacral, solar plexus
Moonstone	Enhances feminine energy, intuition	Sacral, first eye
Blue Agate	Healing, promotes peace of mind	Throat, first eye
Lapis Lazuli	Stimulates higher thoughts, protective	Throat, first eye
Black Tourmaline	Absorbs negative energy, stabilizing	root
Clear Quartz	Healing, energizing, promotes positivity	All
Rose quartz	Promotes divine unconditional love	Heart, all
Lepidolite	Dissipates negativity and electromagnetic pollution, put around computer	Throat, first eye, heart, crown
Amethyst	Promotes spiritual connection, healing	Crown, all
Selenite	Promotes higher guidance, peace	crown

THE PENDULUM

The pendulum is a spiritual tool which shows how to sense or tune in to the subtle energy fields that surround us. The pendulum works by allowing invisible energetic signals to be converted into visible movement through the response of the pendulum. Use of the pendulum is an Ancient technique based on dowsing. If is useful to help make decisions, consult high guidance, develop intuition, and focus the will. In RA SEKHI we use the pendulum to check and balance the aritu and help clear the aura and other energetic blockages.

It can be used to read energy and to program energy as well, that is how it is used to balance and clear the aritu and the aura. You can also use charts with your pendulum to measure things as well. You can judge the energy of something by the speed the pendulum moves and the distance the pendulum swings. Here are basic instructions for using the pendulum :

> *Hold the chain lightly between the thumb and forefinger of the right hand (for incoming information and energy). Hold your hand still and trust the pendulum to move by itself.*
> *Take four deep breaths, relax and go into a meditative state.*
> *Call upon the divine light that is indwelling for guidance to give you clear truthful answers to your questions*

Begin by asking the pendulum to show you (+) yes and (-) no. A clockwise movement is usually positive and counterclockwise is negative. If the pendulum moves vertical or horizontal it is usually negative or no. if the pendulum does not move, relax and think about what you are asking, then try again.

Remember to formulate questions to have yes nor no answers.

Do not ask the same questions over again. Try to remain unbiased when you use your pendulum. remember it is reading your energy, so if you want the answer to come out a certain way, most likely it will.

The more you work with it, the easier it becomes.

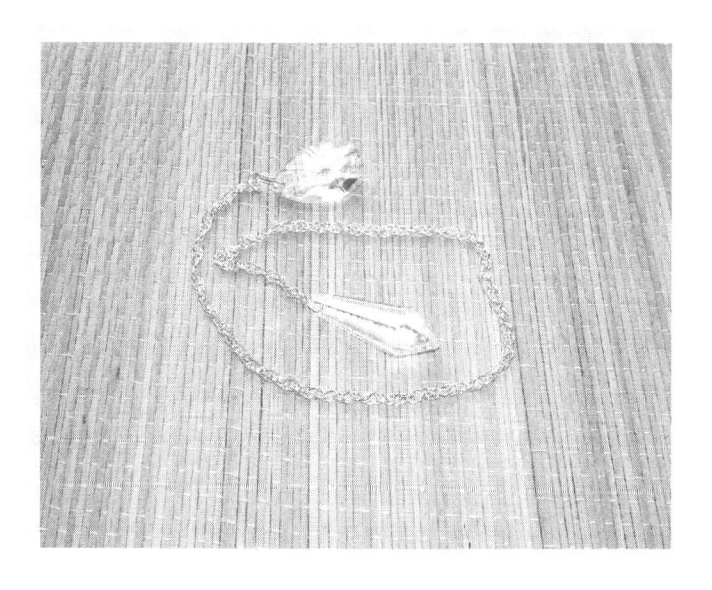

HOW TO RECORD YOUR INITIAL READINGS

Using the BODY DIAGRAM to Record

The Body Diagram has a circle corresponding with each Aritu (Chakra). Use this diagram to mark where your client is stagnant or closed during your scanning and pendulum reading. Write a the letter "C" in the circle where your client is closed and the letter "O" where your client if open. (This will help you keep up with the areas of focus for this session). Use the lines provided to write any additional information you would like to remember about that particular Aritu. This diagram will help you remember the results of your reading during your healing session and will also help you to track your patient's progress over time.

Using the PENDULUM SCALE to Record

Use a scale of 1-10 to determine the level that your client is open or closed. With **1** representing the smallest degree open/closed and **10** representing the largest degree open/closed (a wide swing). For example, if the pendulum is swinging in a very wide circle in the clockwise direction, then most likely to client is between 8-10 degrees open. If the pendulum is swinging in a very small circle in the counterclockwise direction then most likely the client is about 1-3 degrees closed. (The direction and meaning of the swing will be determined when you program your pendulum). If the pendulum does not move at all the client has stagnant energy, which is represented by a **0**. Using this Scale will help you determine your client's needs more accurately.

Clients Name: _____ Date: _____

BODY DIAGRAM

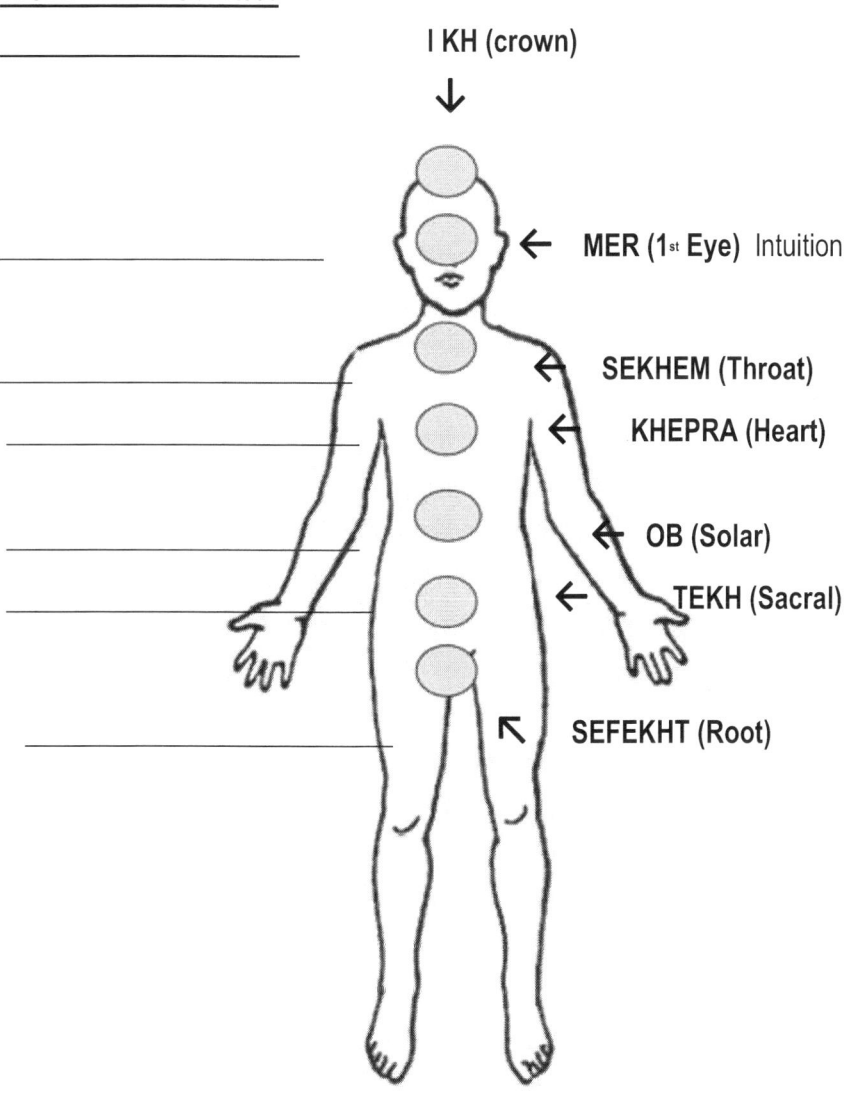

_____

I KH (crown)
↓

← MER (1st Eye) Intuition

← SEKHEM (Throat)

← KHEPRA (Heart)

← OB (Solar)

← TEKH (Sacral)

↖ SEFEKHT (Root)

PENDULUM SCALE

Aritu	Degree Open Scale of (1-10)	Degree Closed Scale of (0-10)
Ikh – 7th		
Mer – 6th		
Sekhem – 5th		
Khepra – 4th		
Ob – 3th		
Tekh – 2nd		
Sefekht – 1st		

NOTE: Please make copies of the charts prior to your session so that you will have them available when it is time to record.

Pendulum Chart

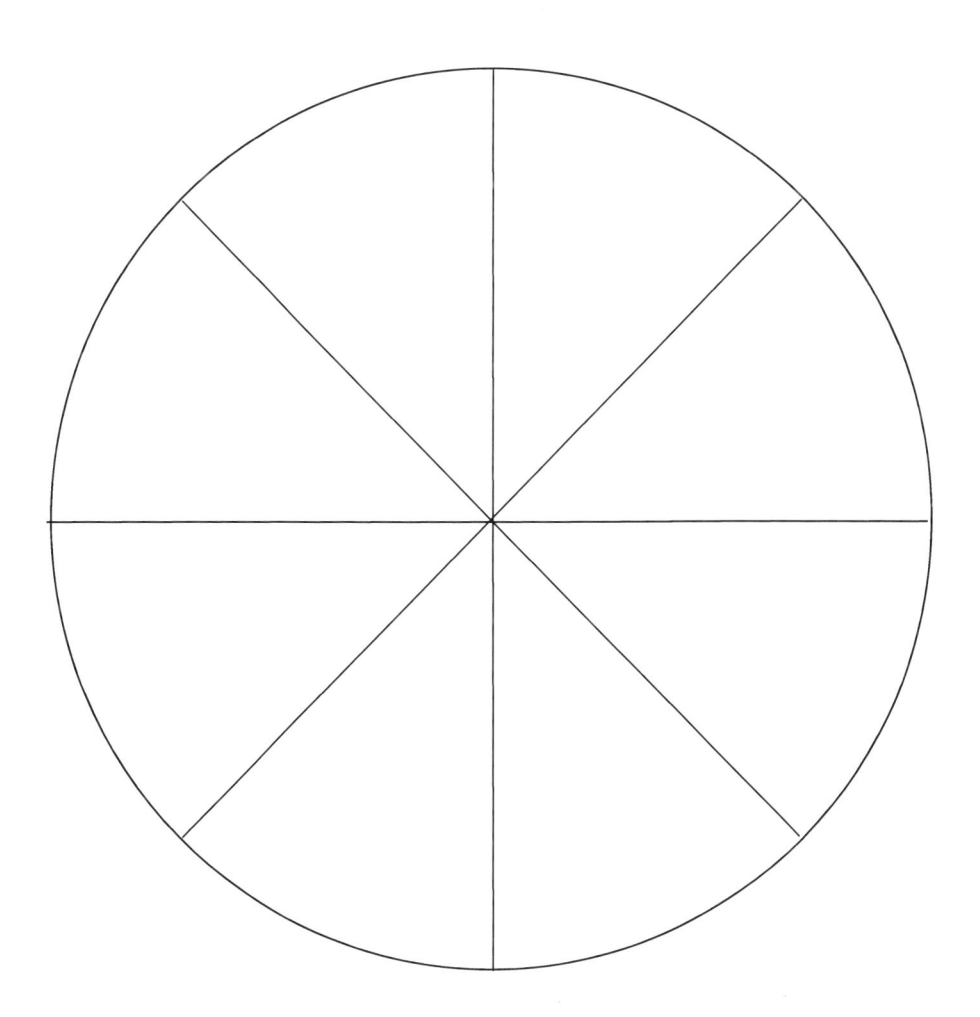

Make copies and use this pendulum chart by adding the names of colors, NTRU, Aritu, etc. for your personal readings.

SPIRITUAL PROTECTION

There are many different spirits on this realm with us right now. Many of them are negative forces and so it is very important that we protect ourselves spiritually from these types of energy. There are levels of negative forces and so the medicine or protection needed depends on the situation. You can be virtually immune from negative influences if you live with good character and don't pollute yourself with the toxins of the world. However since we live on earth and this is a continuous journey ascension we have to take steps to protect ourselves.

You can protect yourself from petty negative vibrations by being mindful of your communication and behavior in your relations. When you create a situation for someone to be mad or upset with you, you can be affected by their thoughts and feelings, especially if your vitality and aura is weak. Creating this type of energy with several people will add up and can cause problems until some resolution is made.

Jealousy and the evil eye are also common forces that we have to protect ourselves from. Usually love energy and overall feeling good can protect you from these energies, however sometimes more powerful things need to be done. There are also talisman (protection pieces) of eyes used and mirrors in the home also protect this kind of negative influence.

Psychic vampires are people who consciously and subconsciously drain your energy. They see your light or sense that you have something they need. They try to tap into your source spiritually and sometime physically and then they begin their work. The best protection for this energy is discernment. You have to be able to recognize what is going on and then cut it short. If it is someone your just meet or see in a store your can immediately leave the environment and begin to chant, pray and put your protection up. Sometimes people we consider friends or lovers can be psychic vampires as well. Once again you have to be aware of the reality of the relationship. Remember as a healer you will attract people who need healing. You have to see these ones as clients and work with them that way. Do not let them get to close and personal with you. Don't allow anyone to drain you of your precious energy without reciprocating in some way. We want to help people without hurting ourselves.

There are much stronger forces that we must also be aware of and be protected from. For these type of forces you want to protect your home, your family and yourself. There are many protective prayers and rituals done . Using candles, protective herbs, symbols on a continuous basis in necessary for the echoes of negative energy is all around at this time. They can come thru radio, TV, media and people. Sea salt, garlic, frankincense, sage, turquoise, tobacco, cinnamon, and coffee are known to have protective energy. Following a lifestyle of MAAT and living in a natural way is the best overall protection. Keep your thoughts, words, actions and your heart pure for you attract more of what you think, say and do.

Here are more helpful tips for protection during healing work.

• Build a protective force field using the RA symbols around yourself. Visualize or use your hands to create a protective force field of symbols.

• We also ask our Spirit Guides for protection before doing a healing session. This is an important step before working on anyone.

• Make a crystal grid as a protective force against negativity. Black stones, clear quartz and citrine are powerful protective stones.

• Wear a clear quartz crystal everyday to help keep your aura strong and clear. Citrine is good as well. Make sure to clean your crystal jewelry often and don't let others touch your jewelry.

• Cover your crown during healing sessions and when going out in crowds or around unfamiliar people.

• Visualize a white or indigo blue flame surrounding you and your family.

Remember your intentions and your good character will add power to your spiritual work. It is important to know that no one has the power to hurt or harm you. When you give in to fear and doubt you open yourself up to allow negative energy to affect you. Do the best you can, do the work and know that you are protected and strong.

Altar Building

As a practitioner you should build an altar as a focal point to communicate with your ancestors. You can start with a personal altar or an ancestral altar. All altars have basic elements that bring the energy together to create a sacred space. You will want to physically clean the area first. Choose and area that in not frequented often in your home. Although different altars have different purposes.

Communication and care of altars spaces help to elevate all parities involved. As we give energy to the Spirit World, they give energy to us. The main elements for altars is to have something to represent

Air- sweeten the air with incense or fragrance when you go there

Fire—light a candle or keep a candle lit on your alter

Water- use a natural container (glass, metal, wood, etc)

Earth—use a plant, container of dirt or crystals

You can use a white cloth for most altars as well.

Personal altar as a place to meditate and do your spiritual work. Personal altars are made to encourage your personal growth and development. Add things that you work with in your healing work , personal books, crystals, instruments, journal, mandala and other spiritual tools. You may also want to add pictures or symbols that make you feel connected to Spirit and to your higher self. You can keep this one in your bedroom or sacred space.

Ancestral Altars are usually close to the ground, so use a low table or put it on the floor. You can use dolls or statues to represent your ancestors. Add other things that remind you of your personal ancestors or pictures. You can also ask what other things they want you to add. Make offerings of food, flowers, song, dance, stories about them, water, tobacco, coffee or tea, etc. Change the water every day on your ancestral altar.

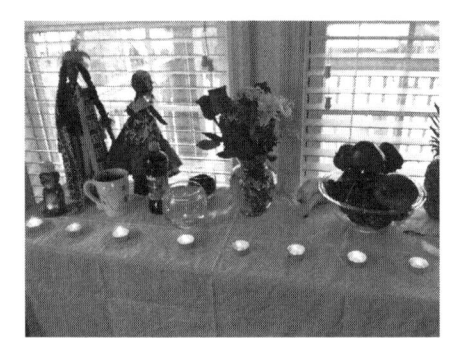

Healing Altar should be in the space where you do your healing work. You can add your healing tools, crystals, instruments, oils, incense, pendulum, etc to this space. A picture of a statue, an ankh and a pyramid are also good to add to your healing altar space.

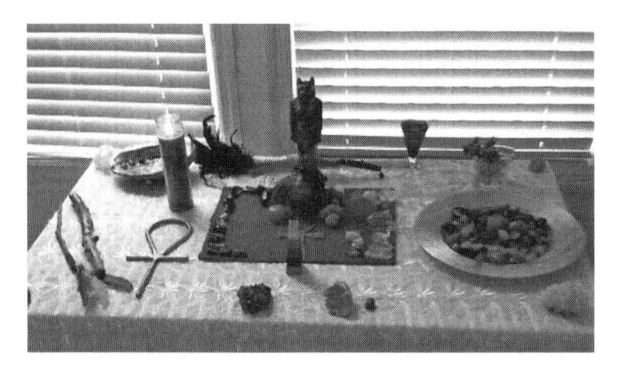

Ra Sekhi Symbols

Ra Sekhi is empowered by the use of symbols. The Sacred symbols are used all over the world to pass the initiation from one to another and to heal. In Ra Sekhi level 1 we learned symbols to work with. Working with them should have developed your ability to focus and concentrate. Level 2 introduces more kemetic symbols but you are not limited to the symbols you can use in your healing work.

Symbols are all around us. Some are universal, some are communal, and some are personal. The Universe is mathematical, and there is specific power in specific lines and shapes. Symbols speak to the soul and can evoke specific thoughts, feelings, and even physical responses. The response can be automatic and unconscious or it can be passionate and intense. Symbols are used in Ra Sekhi to lend us power. There are symbols, which have been used for thousands of years, and when we use them we attract their spiritual presence power and healing tradition.

Many Reiki symbols have been kept very secret until recently. You could not take Reiki II class without first swearing to honor that secrecy. They were originally taught orally, never to be written down. However, that was in a time when every family had their own healer. Times have changed and there is a need for the tradition to continue so the traditional symbols have been printed and put in public view for all those who are interested. Our Ancestors have hundreds of symbols, hieroglyphs, veves and more that have different meanings and have been used for protection, healing, rituals, portals, and similar purposes.

As you memorize symbols, do so precisely. The symbols are living, always in motion and you will learn to use them by inspiration. Practice drawing them in the air, stroke by stroke, repeating their names as you draw. With practice, you'll find that you "see" them settle into place, complete.

The symbols will increase your focus and your depth for healing and they will enable you to do distance healing. The symbols empower you to send healing over distance and time. You can use them over food to cleanse it as you pray. You can use symbols for protection when needed, to bless a room or person.

When sending healing energy to others it is important to ask for permission and honor their free will. You can ask mentally and receive and answer if the person is not physically available. Always use the RA SEKHI symbols and energy for good it is powerless for anything else. Remember karma is real and your intent and energy should reflect pure love (MER) and harmony (MAAT).

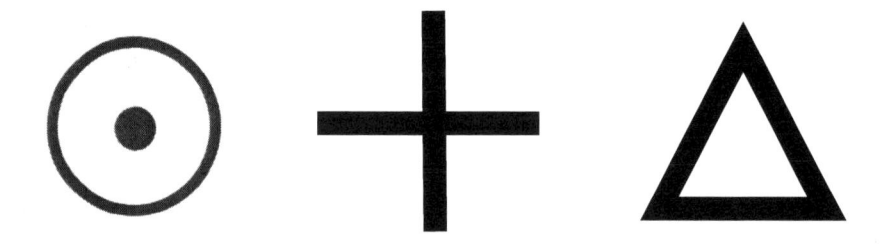

These are universal symbols, known by many names, they represent different aspects of THE MOST HIGH, RA/RAAT, THE SUPREME BEING, LIGHT/SUN POWER, EQUALITY, HIGHER POWER, 360 DEGREES OF WISDOM, THE DIVINE ONE AND ALL. They teach us to focus and balance the right and left hemispheres of the brain. They help to stimulate our inner power. They work to enhance our spiritual connection and connect with intuitive group thinking or the universal consciousness. They can be used for healing and for spiritual protection on individuals and in your environment.

KEMETIC SYMBOLS

ANKH means eternal life, stability and strength. It symbolizes the union of male and female. It is regenerative and a powerful healing symbol used to add vitality and healing energy to ones with imbalance and low vitality.

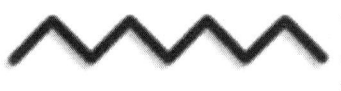

NU/NUN/NUNET means to move about, to find. It is an ancient symbol representing water and lightening. It is purifying and cleansing. It is useful for running energy and adding vitality. It can be used with curved lines, like waves to add more feminine energy.

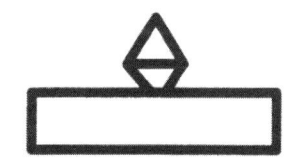

HETEP means peace, content, happy, restful. It symbolizes supreme peace, union with the higher self, and connection with THE SUPREME DIVINE LIGHT. This is the state that we strive to keep at all times. Hetep is useful for a recipient who needs to relax and be calm. It is useful to balance heartache, depression, sorrow, etc... It is also useful to balance someone who is dealing with fiery issues and energy.

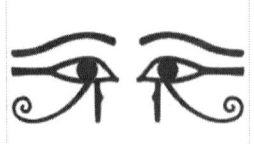

UTCHA means to create, to come forth, to be health, of strength, to protect and "light fiery one." They symbolize the power of NTR, the ability to see all. They are called "THE ALL SEEING EYES" and remind us that all is seen. They help in scanning the recipient to get to the root of the problem. UTCHA can be used like a laser light to bean in on specific areas and will help to identity emotional and spiritual issues that cause physical problems. They will help tap into past lives and their vision is unlimited. It is said that the right eye belongs to RA and the left eye belongs to HERU, this speaks to their fiery, activating and powerful energy.

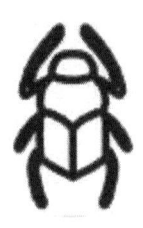

KHEPRA means to be, to make, to come into being, to form, shape, or change. It symbolizes transformation, regeneration, rebirth and growth. It represents the morning sun and is symbolized by a beetle. This symbol is useful for helping to change ones consciousness and to regenerate toxic, dead cells into healthy cells.

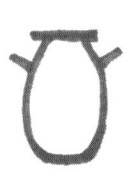

AB means to unite or join together, it is the consciousness of humans and the mother of reincarnation. It represents and is symbolized by the heart. It is the symbol of the unconscious mind, the conscious and unconscious impressions gathered from past and present experiences. It works well with issues of the heart and our Kemetic ancestors would say "My heart, the mother of my coming into being."

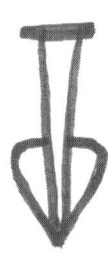

SMA means to bless. It is represented by the union of two lungs and the trachea. It symbolizes the union of the higher and lower self leading to one. It is useful for those who are disconnected from Spirit.

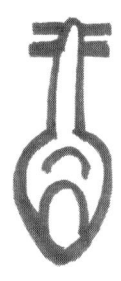

NFR means good, beautiful and happy. It is represented by the union of the heart and trachea. It symbolizes that which is most beautiful, the highest good and the greatest achievement. NFR is close to NRT, nature and THE MOST HIGH. It is useful for those dealing with insecurities, low self-esteem, stress, depression, etc.

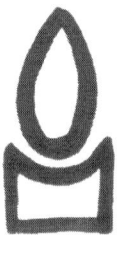

UDJA is the symbol for prosperity, success, fulfillment, strength. It is a good symbol to use at the end of a session to seal and balance the healing energy that was shared. It is also useful for those who need inspiration, motivation, vitality and spiritual strength.

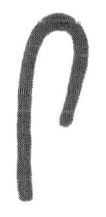

SENEB is the symbol for good health, wellness, strength and to be sound. It brings balance in the emotional, mental, spiritual and physical bodies. Also a good symbol to use at the end of the healing session to promote overall health and wellness to the client.

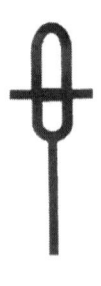

SEKHEM is the life force energy or power that exist within the universe. The symbol of Sekhem is represented by the hand held staff. It refers to a scepter that means physical power, authority, and strength. Sekhem is the Spiritual personification of the vital life force in humans, all life draws upon this force in order to exist. It is useful to use in all dis-eases of all

Non-Traditional Reiki Symbols

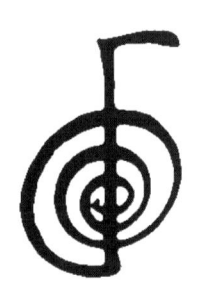

Cho Ku Rei "I am calling all the power of the universe"

Cho a curved line, **Ku** penetrating to make whole, a whirlwind spiral, **Rei** Universal Soul, Spirit, Essence.

CkR is a circular shape representing the conch shell, symbolizing the calling of The Higher Power. It penetrates, empower, and is used for transformation and transition. This symbol resonates with the physical body. It is a power symbol and multiplies energy, like turning on a light bulb. It invokes the Universal Life Energy and love to NTR. It comforts and balances the recipients and blesses them, increasing their good. Use it in difficult situations to bring blessings. Use clockwise to open and expand, counterclockwise to close and contract.

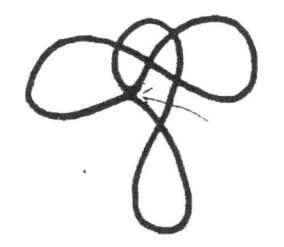

SE HE KI "I AM THE HIDDEN BALANCE"

SE things hidden inside, the origin of external form, HEKI the hidden balance, life force energy

SHK is used to balance the upper four chakras for mental, emotional, and spiritual balancing and cleansing. It goes to the root of mental problems, emotional balances, and addictions of any kind. It is the symbol for emotional holding and subconscious. It is the pattern breaker and aligns our mental and emotional bodies with Divine Spirit. It assists us in removing block from the flow of energy, opens and protects the recipient. It calls on Divine Healers or Angelic power for assistance.

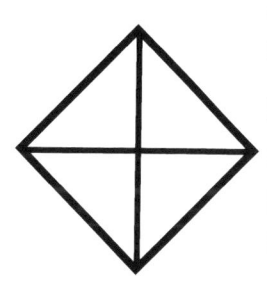

HON SHA SE SHO NEN "I AM SHIMMERING ESSENCE ADVANCING ON TARGET"

HON center, origin, start, nature. SHA shimmering light ze advancing, moving ahead, SHO target, enlightening, integrity, NEN stillness, thinking in the deepest part of the mind.

HSZSH unifies time and space, giving us understanding of distance healing. It acts as an ether tube connecting for sending distance-healing energy. This symbol works on the mental body. It empowers the recipient to get in touch with her Higher Spirit. It also invokes the Karmic healing of a lineage and is about manifesting wellness.

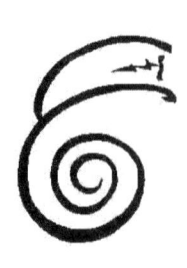

DAI KOO MYO "I RADIATE THE ALL PERMEATING LIGHT OF THE ENLIGHTENED ONES"

DAI big, magnificent, expansive, KOO radiance, fire or light expansion at the crown chakra, MYO clairvoyance, green light piercing thru earthly planes beyond phenomenon, divine wisdom

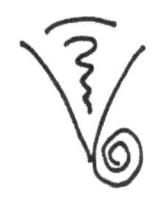

DKM works on the spiritual level. It is an "I am" symbol, the Law of One, saying, "God in me heals." It focuses on healing the soul and the heart chakra sending Divine Love. It heals the first cause of dis-ease, making life changes. These are two versions of the same symbol.

The Asian symbols are known to work very well, however we know Afrikan symbols are more familiar to Afrikan people and will work more specifically with us. There are said to be over 400 Reiki symbols of which 22 were commonly used. These symbols we presented are ones that we know to work, however other symbols may be used in your practice. Right now there are many new symbols being used because some are too Oriental and difficult to learn. The new symbols work directly with the Divine work that is taking place on Earth at this time.

Ra Sekhi Healing Sessions

Before you begin to do healing work make sure that you have practiced on yourself and family members. This will give you some experience in working with energy outside of your own. When you feel comfortable about working with others you can begin to look for a space, in a massage studio or beauty salon. You can also begin to see clients in your home. Make sure that you use a particular room that is not used often by family members if possible. Also it is good to have an altar in your healing space as well.

Be sure to add natural elements fire , air, water and earth. Candles, soft lights, soft music, plants, crystals, fountains and other natural elements help to maintain balance in your healing space. You will want to keep the space physically and spiritually clean. Burn incense, open windows and doors, pray chant and sing in the space often to help keep things clear and moving.

You can use a massage table, Afrikan slant chair or other comfortable chair for your clients to sit on. It is important that the client is comfortable while receiving the healing energy.

It is good to begin with smudging the client before they sit down. You may also want to have your crystal grid set as well. Remember to prepare yourself with deep breathing or fire breathes. You may also want to fast and prepare yourself with healing sessions before working on someone else.

Say a pray before the client arrives then again once they are seated. You can help them relax with a meditation or deep breathing exercise.

Before you start say a prayer to call your Spirit Guides to help you and ask for protection. Begin the healing session by putting your hands first over the clients crown aritu. This is how you make contact with them. Take a few minuets to feel the energy and notice what you feel.

Next begin to scan the clients energy, begin at the crown and move slowly down the persons body. Make sure to notice any changes in their energy. You may feel a cold area, then some are areas that is warm. Determine which area needs extra attention, tune in to hear any messages that may come.

Next, begin to sweep the clients aura. Start from the top of their head and move down to the feet. This time move your hands faster as if they are sweeping like a broom would. Visualize you clearing any blockages the client may have. Make sure you clear away as much as possible.

The next step is to check the aritu. Use the pendulum over each aritu and ask if they are open, balanced or active. The aritu that are unbalanced will need some extra attention to get reactivated. You can start this process by laying a coordinating crystal on the aritu

After placing crystals on your clients use sound therapy to initiate positive changes, to clear blockages and to continue to clear the aura. Swinging a bell or rattle directly over a blocked aritu is an outstanding way to bring healing and balance to those areas. Different sounds work differently for everyone so ask your Spirit Guides to help you determine what your client needs. When you feel you have cleared the aura and removed blockages adequately, you can proceed to the palm healing.

Start at the crown arit and work you way down your clients body with hand positions. Take extra time in those special areas that you noticed during you scan. While doing palm healing you can sing, chant, pray or be quiet. You can visualize certain colors, symbols or other healing image in your mind as you go through the clients body. Your hands do not have to touch your client, the energy will flow if they are next to you or across the world.

When you are finished the healing work, you can seal your client in a golden or white light bubble. The bubble will work to keep the healing energy flowing to your client and circulating within their energy field. Also make sure to put your hands on the bottom of the clients feet to ground them. At this time you can also thank the spirit guides who came forth to work with you.

You can speak to your client while doing the work on them, be mindful that they may drift off into sleep or astral travel while you are working on them.

Energy Scanning is done with you hands. When you place you hands over someone for the first time you are making contact with their aura and energy. Take time to feel the energy, then begin moving slowly over their auric field. Notice the areas that feel different, you may feel a coolness or more heat in these areas. Continue to move down to the persons feet. You can revisit the trouble spots again and ask what is needed to balance these areas.

Chakra Balancing is done in a variety of ways. You want to read the aritu with your hands or pendulum to find if they are active, balanced or unbalanced. You can hold the pendulum directly over the arit and ask if it is open. notice the direction and the rate the pendulum moves. If the pendulum moves in a negative swing the aritu is unbalanced most likely. You may notice the pendulum swing in the same or they could swing in different directions. The pendulum also may not move at all which usually means there is blockage in that area. Your reading should be in alignment with your energy scan.

Adding crystals to the unbalanced arit will assist in the balancing process. You can also use the pendulum to direct the arit to swing in a positive direction. You can use different instruments directly over blocked areas to dissipate the blockage and promote positive energy flow.

Also using your hands with symbols and color visualization is very powerful to balance the arit. Focus your energy on MAAT and balance as you do this.

Aura cleansing is important to do before doing palm therapy. When we clear ones aura, we may feel negative energy and we must use our intentions and visuals to help dissipate the energy. You can visualize the energy going into the floor and into the earth, or out into the universe to be transformed into something else. Using hand claps or sudden noise and certain baths or herbs also help to clear negative energy off of one.

Florida water, holy water or spiritual bath should be used often as a practitioner to help you stay light and focused and may be used during a healing session as well. After the session clear the space with holy water, blessed broom and prayers to dissipate all that was released from the client. It is also helpful to take a spiritual bath after doing work on others as well. Do all you can to clear others energy off of you.

Become sensitive enough to your own energy so you will know when you need to clear others energy off of you. People who do physical work with others, like massage therapists, beauticians, pedicurists, colon therapists, etc. Should also take extra precaution to clear their energy on a regular basis. Remember energy can build up in layers and one can carry layers of negative energy for years without knowing it. However at some point these layers will lead to dis-ease in some form in the physical body.

The energy will work to heal and balance the emotional, mental, spiritual and physical bodies. Healthy eating and living habits will contribute to the overall healing and well being of the client. Miracles do happen, but we take the approach of doing all that we can to bring about balance within, especially if one is dealing with serious health issues. The more serious the issue is, the more energy healing sessions you will need to truly balance your client. Remember as a healer you want to learn as much as you can to be the best healer you can. People have a variety of health issues to deal with, and everything does not work for everybody.

Practitioner Hand Positions

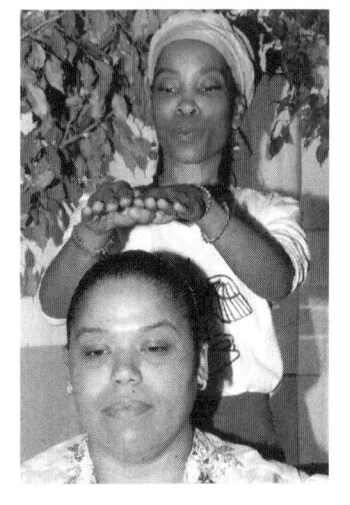

IKH/CROWN

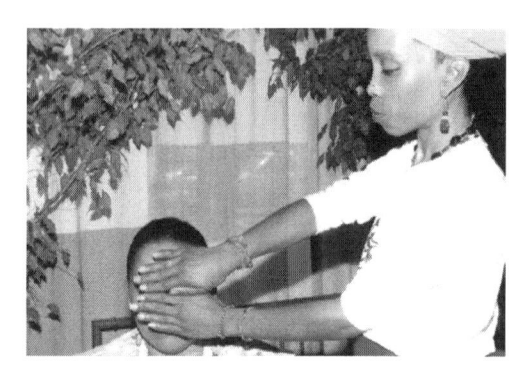

MER/1ST EYE

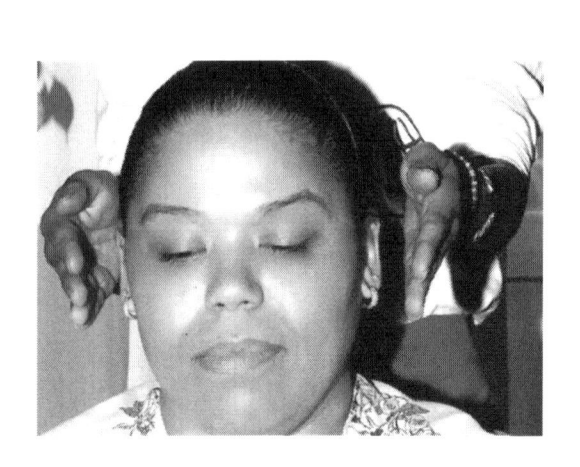

PITUITARY GLAND

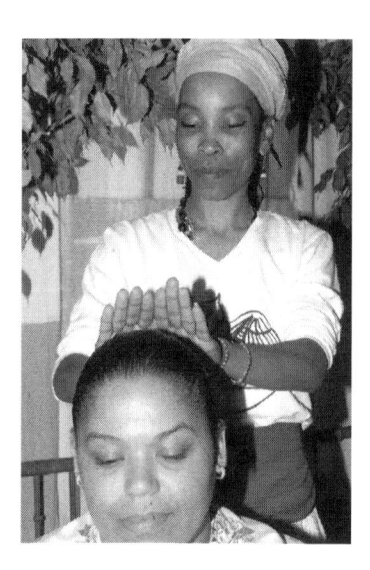

PINEAL GLAND

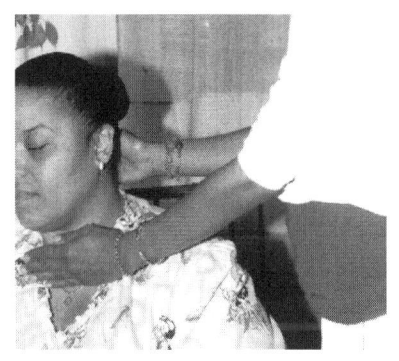

SEKHEM/THROAT

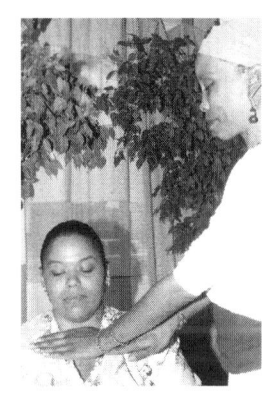

HIGH HEART

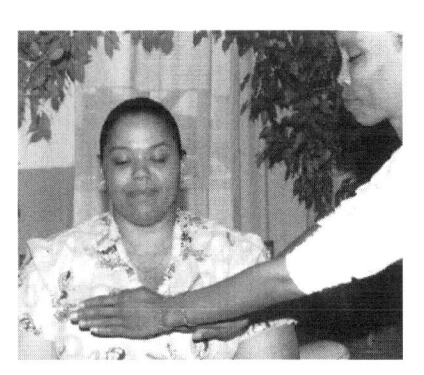

KHEPERA/HEART

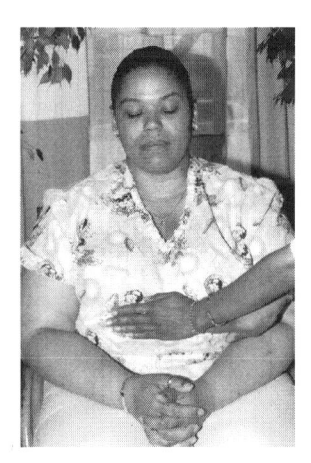

OB/SOLAR PLEXUS

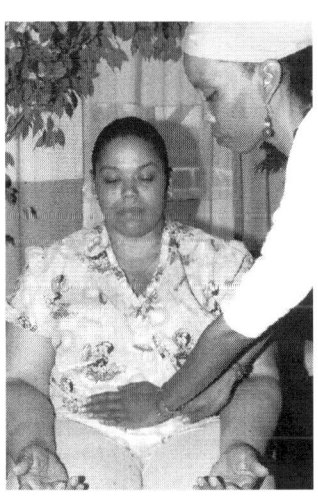

TEKH/SACRAL
& SEFKHET/ROOT

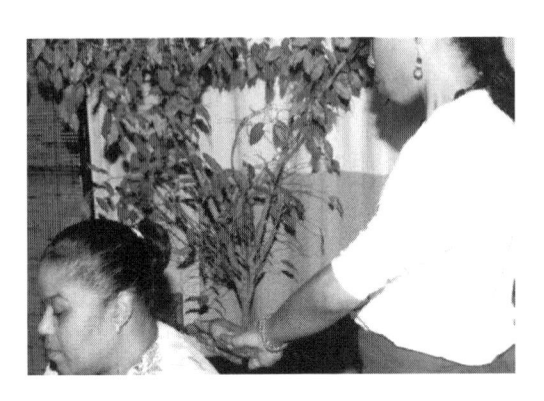

KHEPERA/HEART

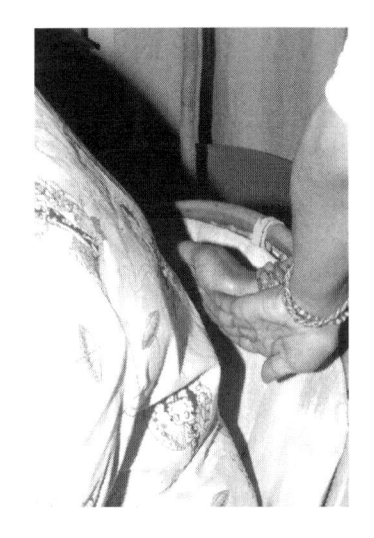

OB/SOLAR PLEXUS

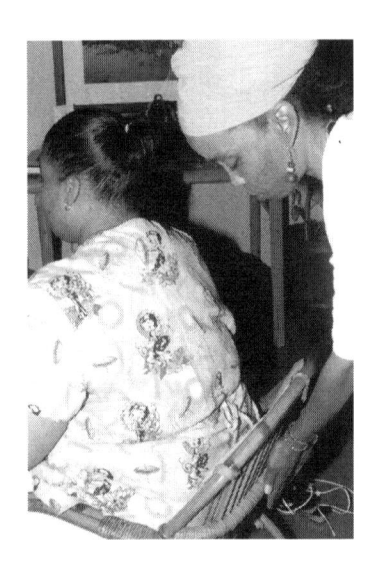

TEKH/SACRAL & SEFKHET/ROOT

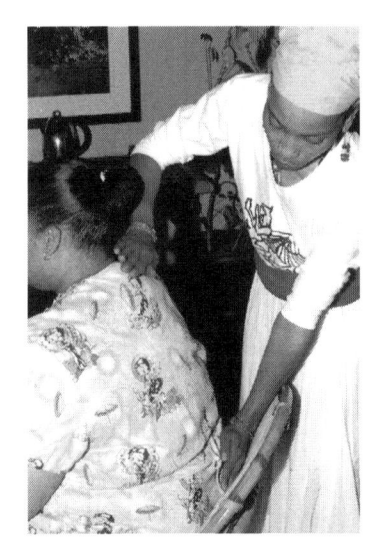

BALANCING SEKHEM THRU ARITU

MINOR ARITU

MINOR ARITU

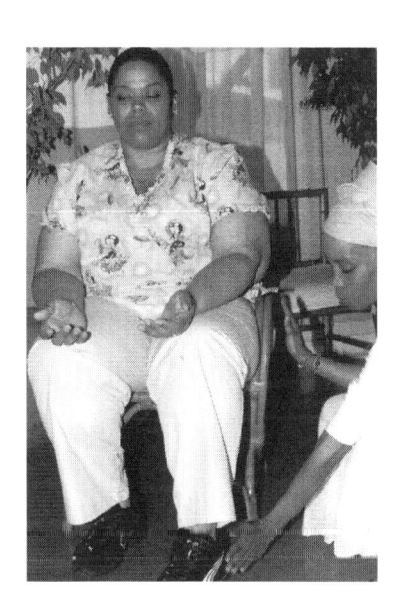

RUNNING SEKHEM
THRU ARITU

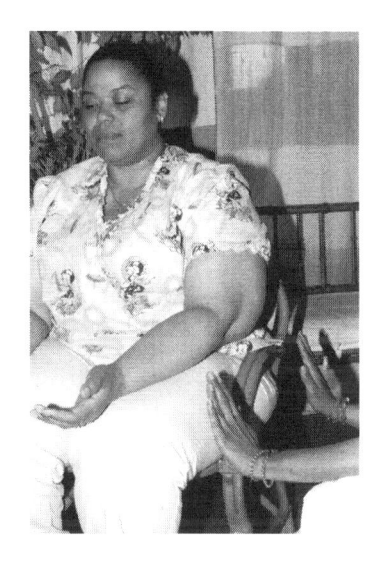

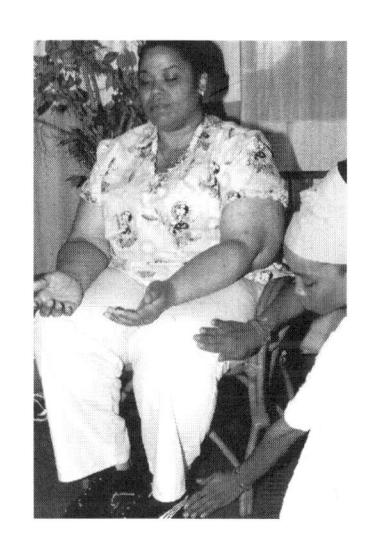

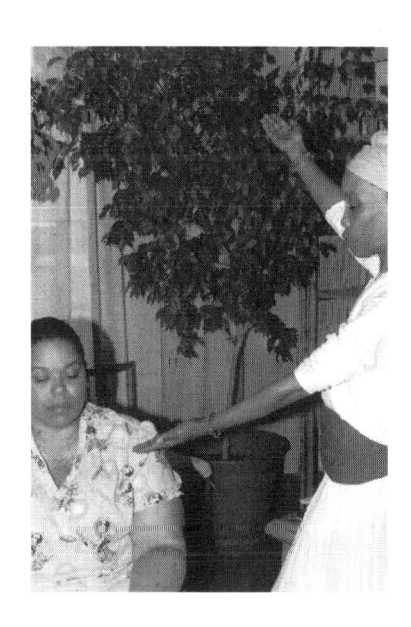

CHANNELING PURE
LIGHT ENERGY

55

Group Healing

Group Healing is an opportunity for one to receive a great amount of energy at one time. In fact everyone involved in the healing receives benefits from these healing sessions. Group healing sessions are especially helpful for those who have serious health issues like cancer, tumors, diseases of the immune system, etc. It is important for those in the group to be in tune with each other so the session moves smoothly, and has a good flow. Usually everyone helps to clear the aura of the client. Then one or two may check the aritu and do energy scanning.

Next everyone assumes a position usually one on each side of the person. If there are more than two healers, ones can also work at the head and feet. Two to four healers at a time is usually a good balance for one client.

Healers may move around in a circle during the session and change positions. Make sure to move in a way that will not disturb the healing. Chant together and work together for the betterment of the client, You can also stand outside of the circle and send energy and prayers with hands in a ka position.

You will feel the energy rise during the beginning of the session and then it will subside. At that time healers should make sure that everyone is ready to close. Check the aritu before you close to make sure they are balanced. Then ground the client and give thanks to the Spirit Guides for the healing energy.

Group Healing

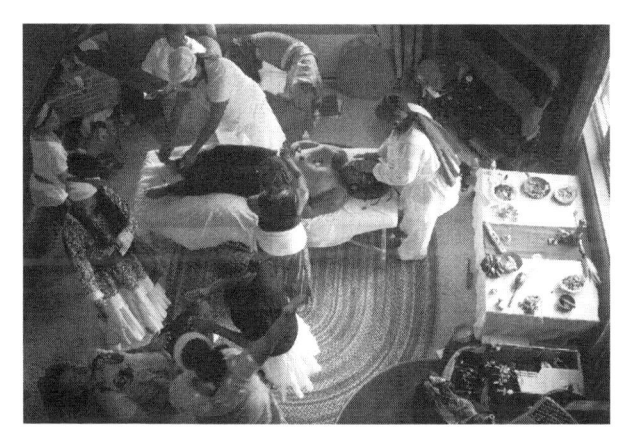

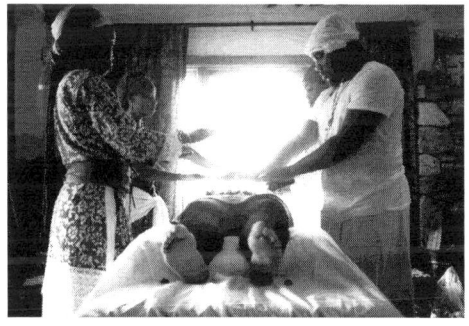

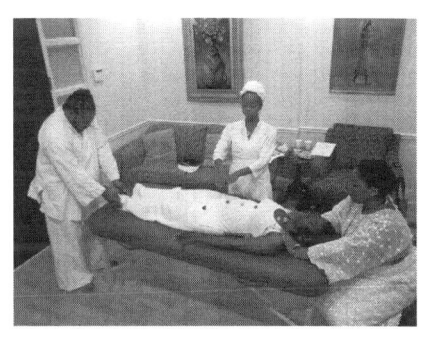

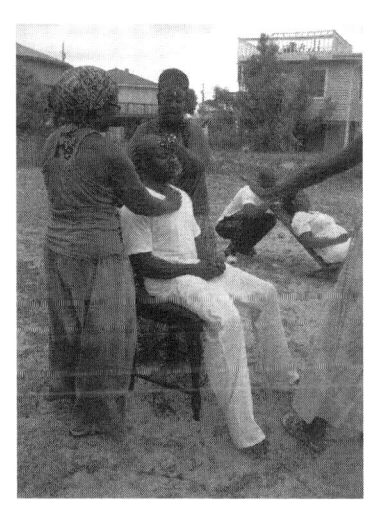

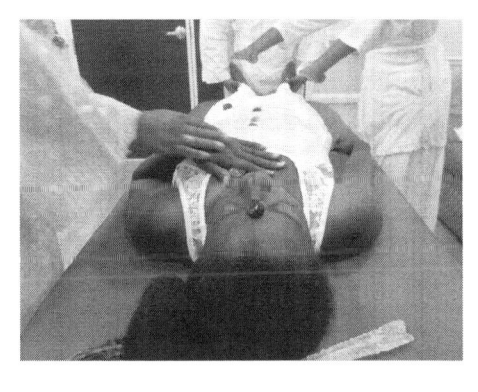

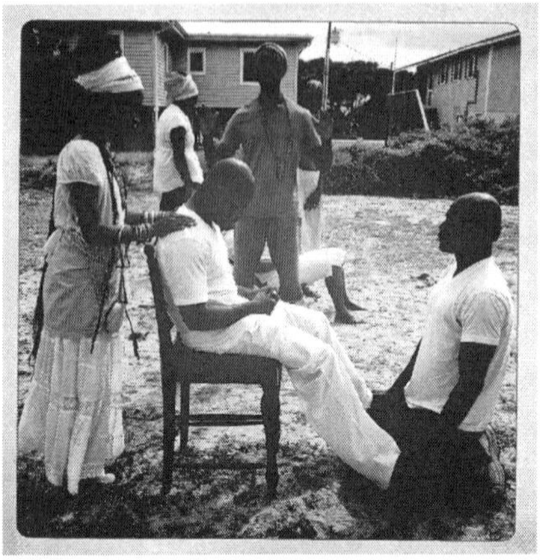
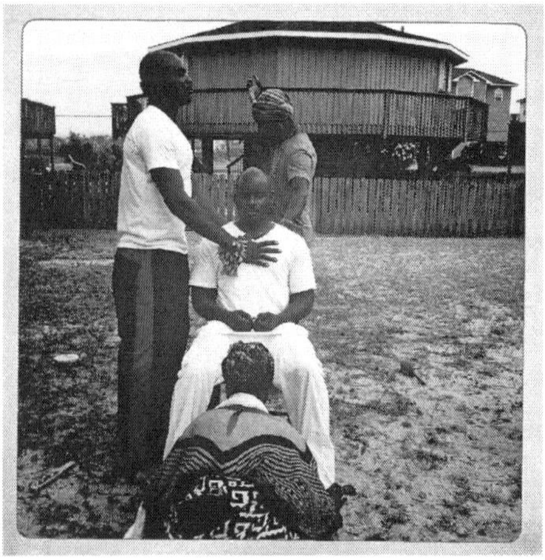
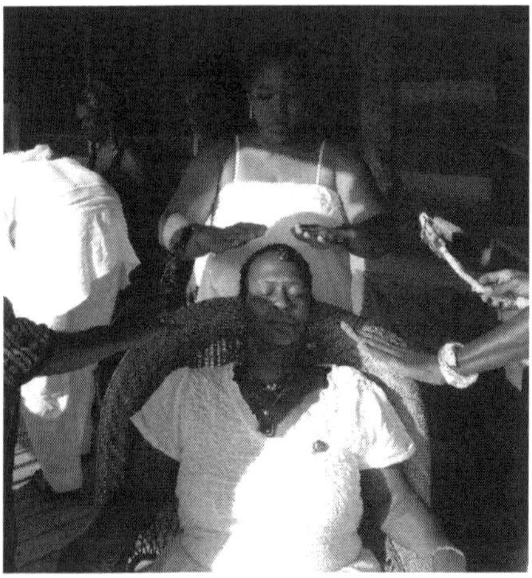
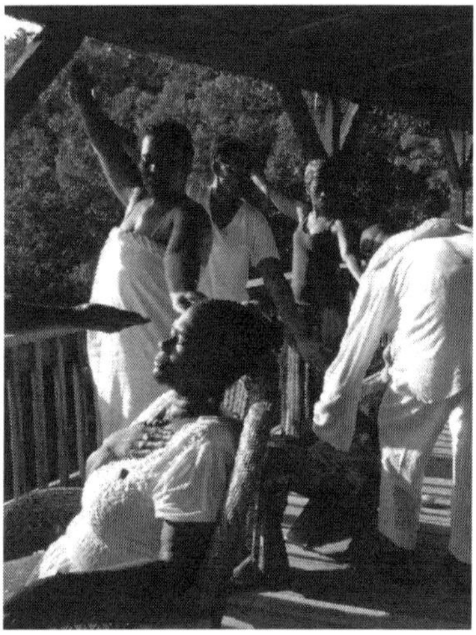
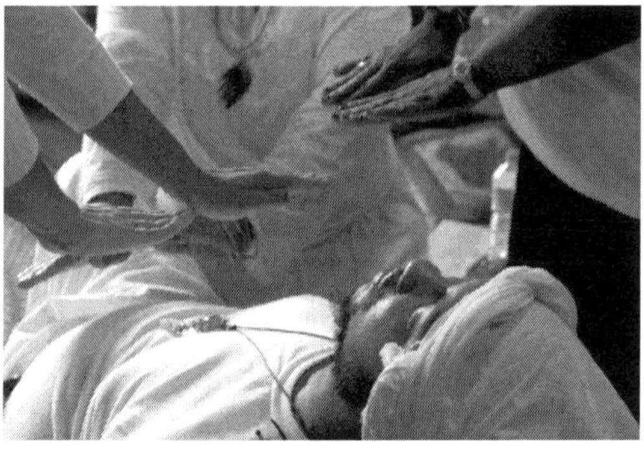

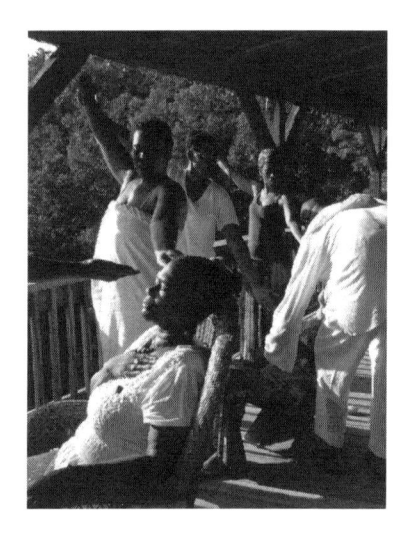

Release Ritual

This releasing ritual is best done with a group. We all have things that we have been carrying and this ritual will bring relief to that weight energetically and spiritually. You begin with smudging the client and seating them in a comfortable chair. Then you want to take them through a guided meditation to help them relax. Then you begin clearing the aura with the hands with someone on each side of the client. The one behind the client will act as leader in the ritual. They will place their hands on the clients shoulders and begin speaking. Take your time going thru each sentence and give the client an opportunity to release. When you begin the aura cleansing start with light and gentle strokes. The energy and the clearing usually picks up as you continue. Instruments, chanting and continuous clearing is necessary.

Release the pain from your childhood.

Release any pain from your teenage years.

Release any pain or anger you may be feeling.

Release any sadness or doubts you may feel.

Release any guilt or worries you may have.

Release any pain from past lifetimes you may have..

Release any pain from past relationships you may be holding.

Release any negative emotions or blockages you may feel.

Release all that is not serving your highest good.

Now ask the client to speak and verbally release their personal thoughts and feelings. Give them as much time as they need. They may cry at any time during this ritual so it is good to have tissue ready and be responsive to the person's needs. Make sure your send the energy you are clearing out of an window or door. You may also have to use your hands or visualization to cut ties during this session as well.

When the client is ready as them if they are ready to stand up. Then ask them to repeat this mantra

As I heal myself I heal my children

As I heal myself I heal my family.

As I heal myself I heal my community.

As I heal myself I heal the world.

Then ask them to turn around 3 times to the right and say *I am free.... I am free .... I am free*

Make sure to smudge and clear each healer after this session. Also clear the space and give thanks to the Spirit Guides. Make a crystal grid around the healer chair before you start. Quartz crystal, amethyst and black stones work well.

Distance Healing

RA SEKHI can be used to heal one who is not physically present. We can also heal our past and future live with energy healing. Energy transcends time and space, therefore with the right tools and the right energy one can effectively send healing energy to another, and the receiver will feel the energy just as they should.

It is very important that you build up your sekhem before doing distance healing. It also takes a great amount of focus and concentration to send energy to someone who is not in front of you. However it does work in beautiful ways. Sometimes it is helpful to use a doll or draw a picture of a person that you use only for your distance healing sessions. Using a picture of the person you are working on in helpful. You also want to know their full name and birthdate to make a connection with their energy directly.

Begin with creating a healing space

Do several fire breaths then do the sun salutation to raise your sekhem. Raise your hands above your head and connect with Ra/Raat and your Spirit Guides. Chant Ankh three times.

Visualize your healing symbols and send them into your energy field through your Crown chakra. Project the images out into the ethers.

Ask for assistance by calling your Spirit Guides/Neteru/ Orisha/Abosom. Ask them to protect you while doing the work. Ask them to work with you and thru you. Ask that the work be done for the highest good of your client and yourself.

Say mentally or aloud the name of the person who is to receive healing you may also use a drawing or picture.

Visualize the symbols for Ra and make connection with the client. Honor their spirit within and thank them for the opportunity to work with them.

Ask what is the problem and wait for an answer

Picture them laying in front of you and proceed to give the healing as if they were there.

When finished surround them with gold light. Thank them and the Spirit Guides for the healing work they have done.

Release the healing space

You should set an appointment for your distance healing session. You and the client should be in a quiet and peaceful place during the session. The client can sit or lay down in a comfortable position. If it is not possible or there is and emergency situation you can send energy healing anytime. Follow the steps as closely as possible and know that you have the power to do the work anywhere and anytime.

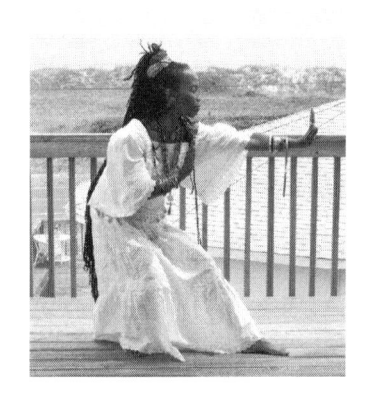

Ra Sekhi Procedures

- Treat yourself daily, add Ra Sekhi to your morning ritual, work on self, and do affirmations.
- The client must make a verbal agreement to participate.
- Wash your hands before and after giving a treatment. Also be conscious of your hygiene, you will have close contact with your client.
- To ensure the free flow of energy be sure the client does not cross their legs or arms during a healing session. Also remove clients' glasses or tight accessories.
- Let your client know that Ra Sekhi does not end when the session does. The energy will continue to flow for days after
- Never diagnose unless you are licensed to do so. Use words like you can share, help, or assist in balancing dis-ease, rather than cure.
- Keep your fingers together when doing a healing session, scattered fingers are scattered energy. Keep hands touching each other unless necessary.
- When changing positions keep gentle contact with the client body or aura.
- Hands can be 1 to 5 inches over the client's body only touch if guided to do so.
- Cleanse the room before and after giving a treatment. Use incense, essential oil (frankincense, sage, etc) crystals and symbols, florida water and/or salt water.

♦ Encourage client to adopt a health lifestyle (eating habits, exercise, etc). this will assist the healing process and help maintain balance.

♦ Provide a quiet healing environment with comfortable chair or massage table. Meditative music, soft lights, candles, and colors are helpful as well.

♦ Have a blanket available as the body temperature may drop with relaxation, also keep tissue handy.

♦ Center yourself before beginning, connect with THE HIGHER POWER within you and the client dedicated each session to the highest good for client and yourself.

♦ After healing session let the client remain quiet and still as long as they need to.

♦ The speed of healing and number of sessions depend on the clients participation, they are the final authority as to when the energy is balanced.

♦ RA SEKHI sessions activate a detoxing process so therapist and clients must drink more water to flush the toxins out of the system.

♦ For maximum healing results, give full treatments for 3 or 4 consecutive days, then 3 sessions the next week, 2 the next week, then 1 the fourth week and then as needed. Group healing sessions are known to speed the healing process. Also RA SEKHI Attunement for someone in the household of the client is helpful for some issues.

♦ When you give a RA SEKHI session the energy will fill you before it flows from your hands, so you receive healing with every healing session you do. "AS YOU GIVE YOU RECEIVE." Your mind, emotions, or physical body

- You are not in control of the healing, Remember to Give Thanks to THE MOST HIGH and the SPIRIT GUIDES, NETERU, ORISHA, ABOSOM, and the ANCESTORS for healing energy and wisdom after each session.

After taking RA SEKHI II it is important to work on yourself, then on family and friends. After doing this you will gain the experience and confidence to share with others as a practitioner. Using RA SEKHI will heal and bring Divine balance to your life, as well as some enlightening spiritual experiences. The most important thing is the quality and strength or your intention. You need to align yourself with the nature of RA SEKHI. Your Spirit Guides will work with you as long as you don't try to use it in a negative way. You should receive an exchange of energy for your service, ask your Spirit Guides for assistance. You may also exchange RA SEKHI with other therapists, offer a free RA SEKHI evening, give healing to people at a gathering. You will be holding a great amount of energy so remember to share with others, with animals, plants, and whenever needed.

Also remember that you are working with the Universe to assist your client the best you can. Sometimes this brings the desired result, sometimes not. You can only do your best, follow your Spirit Guides and keep yourself protected. It is up to your client and the The Most High to determine their fate. Therefore do not take it personal when one does not heal the way you think they should. It is not for you to heal everyone. Always give thanks for the healing and miracles that do happen.

Ra Sekhi Practitioner Protocol

These standards are set to help you raise and cultivate your sekhem. Use this time to learn to work with energy. Share energy healing with others. Study and use the tools you have learned. Begin the process of reclaiming your culture and healing traditions.

Your practice is key to your work. Practice sound therapy, color therapy, crystal therapy, palm therapy, breathing, meditation, affirmations, communication with Spirit Guides and prayers

Wear white or light colors when doing healing work. Also keep your head covered during healing sessions.

Do healing work on yourself 3-4 times a week.

Exercise 3-4 times a week.

Transform your eating habits to vegan (no meat products, do not eat anything that can crawl, walk swim or fly)

Stay in contact with the group via phone calls or email

Do not shake hands or deal with items that are unclean if possible (ie trash), keep your hands clean.

Set up your practice to see clients.

Volunteer to do healing work on elders and children regularly.

Participate in Ra Sekhi healing circles /shares.

Cleanse and fast regularly

Contribute to the Ra Sekhi Temple in some way

Have regular consultations and readings with Snwt.

Work with Sekhmet on Tues, Fri and Sun.

Do not discuss Temple business with those outside of the temple.

Live according to the laws of MAAT therefore there should be no gossiping, lying or other ill behavior. When you give your word you are expected to honor it.

Honor yourself and your Spiritual family at all times.

Dua NTR   Dua SEKHMET

Hygiene and Appearance

Cleanliness is next to Godliness. This is an old proverb that stands the test of time. It is said that the high Spirits will not even come to a person or home that is not clean. In our practice we do practice the art of cleanliness of our bodies and our environment. Before doing any spiritual or healing work you should make sure to clean your body. Ancient Kemetic Priests were known to bath twice a day to remain clean and keep negativity away. Cleaning the mouth, nose, eyes and ears are just as important as a healer. You should take the time to rinse these areas before prayers or healing work.

Another practice of our ancestors is to oil yourself with fragranced oil. Take the time to give yourself a gentle body massage from head to toe with fragranced shea butter. This will add to your overall health, especially if .you use essential oils. Choose Rose, lavender, frankincense or other high vibration oil. Also remember that when you deal with any spiritual work it is always important to dress well in clean and nice clothing. You are going before great forces and as a channel for the energy you are representing or magnifying the God force within you. Your outside appearance should reflect that. Take the time to connect with and enhance your natural beauty . The Spirit Guides love to work with a beautiful and confident being.

Your home and work space should also be free clutter, dust and dirt. If you keep altars in your home you must also make sure your keep the house physically and spiritually clean and clear. Shift or move your furniture to get into spaces that are missed. Organize your closets and drawers. Keeping order in your home is part of living in MAAT. It will help to keep your family and your energy more balanced. Use plants, colors, crystals, water fountains, Afrikan pictures and statues to decorate and keep the energy high in your home. Invite the High Spirits to dwell with you.

Setting up your practice

This book is a manual for Ra Sekhi practitioners. If you have not taken a class with a certified Ra Sekhi Teacher, you cannot call yourself a Ra Sekhi practitioner. However for those who do practice healing work, feel free to use this book as an addition to your practice. Energy healing is serious work. It should not be taken lightly, nor should one jump into doing this work without guidance from Spirit Guides, mentor, elder or teacher.

Before you can truly call yourself a healer you have to heal yourself. You have to know how the energy feels, learn to listen to your intuition and Spirit Guides, learn to work with the colors and symbols. Next you work on those who are close to you. Those you live with, you close friends and extended family members are important to work with. You can watch their progress and changes as you continue the work and learn valuable lessons about moving energy. Also as you change and shift you want to share the positive changes with your household and this will make things more smooth for everyone in the end. They may protest to trying new things but once they feel the good energy they will usually go with it.

As you are practicing on your family begin to thing about your practice. Think of a name for your healing business, something that reflects your energy. Think about where you are set up your healing business. Many times people work from their homes to start with to keep expenses low. Building up your clients takes time so working from your home will allow you time to do this without adding expenses. If you have a room in your home that you can devote to your work that is best. You want to have a space that is quiet, clean, and peaceful. Remember to clear the energy in your home weekly if you are working there so others energy will not effect your household.

If you cannot work from home you may want to see if you can rent a space in a wellness center, yoga studio, health food store, or rent a small office space. Working near someone who already has customers or client who appreciate alternative healing will be helpful. Marketing, promotions and advertising is key. Usually this is a challenge for those of us who are spiritual, but if we are flexible and open we can have a successful business too.

Business cards are important because you want to have a means for people to connect with you. You can order cards online or at your local office/copy store. You can make flyers or a brochure to share your info and to hand out at events around your area. Also hang your flyers in bookstores, health food stores, and other business in your area so people will know what you are doing.

You may also want to set up a website. There are many sites you can use to set up your own site for free. They have templates which make it very easy to do. You an also buy a .com for your site which makes it easier for people to get to you. There are also many people who will create a website for you for a price, usually ranging between $200= $800 depending on what you want on your site.

Doing mini sessions, aura cleansing, chakras balancing, etc at events is another good way to let people know what you do. If you ask event coordinator for a small space to set up your chair or massage table , you should get a lower price then those who are just selling items. Make sure to take a sign with the services you are offering to post near you. Keep in mind where you are going and who your audience will be, everyone may not be ready to see a

When you start working with others you want to think about the services you are going to offer. Usually alternative healers have a base price of $1 per minute for services. Some services may require more energy then others so you can adjust your prices accordingly. You can also look at others in your area who are doing similar work and see what they are charging to give you an idea of what people are paying for alternative healing in your area. There should be some exchange of energy when you share your healing light. You can barter or exchange services or items as well. For clients who have serious problems and may need a series of healing sessions you may want to adjust your price to fit the situation. We try not to turn down anyone who asks for help even if they cannot afford our services. We are here to serve the community and we should know that all that we give will come back to us.

You should do healing work because you love it, not for financial gain. Keep your heart in the right place and it will go well for you. The important thing is to start. If you have taken a class to become a practitioner you want to use your energy and avoid any karmic influence of not stepping into it. Know that you can heal with your presence, your words, your thoughts, your hug and your touch. Be a healer in every moment and take the opportunities that open up to you. Share and teach people about what you are doing, what it has done for you, and why you are doing it. Ra Sekhi and energy healing is new to our community in this time, so how we present it and what we do is key to how our people will receive it and how it will affect our community. Our work is to uplift and heal and we have to keep that in mind all the time. We have to teach while we heal and it can happen in a grocery store, at your office, a PTA meeting, the post office, etc. True healing occurs when one is ready to be healed. When Spirit sees that you are ready, people will begin to call you or catch your attention to discuss their problems. These are your clients. Be prepared to work with them and use all that you know. Do your best, look your best, keep your energy high and know that you are moving with Divine Spirit.

Following are prayers you can use before healing sessions or spiritual work. Feel free to create your own, the power of prayer is infinite.

ANKH UDJA SENEB

GUIDE ME & HEAL ME SO I MAY BE OF GREATER SERVICE TO OTHERS. MAY ALL AVAILABLE HEALERS PLEASE ASSIST ME IN BECOMING A PURE CHANNEL FOR LOVING RA SEKHI ENERGY AND PROVIDE ME WITH THE PROTECTION I NEED. SO IT IS TUA NTR

Bless my hands that they may tools of healing light.

Bless my thoughts that I may be in alignment with the divine. Bless my mouth that my words are of healing and kindness. Bless my Heart that my actions are full of love. Bless this healing session that it may be for the highest good of us all

Ashe amen ra Maat

I am that I am

I am a shining being of light

I aks that only the highest good for all happens here

So it is. Tua ntr

Closing devotional prayer of aspirants

Amma su en pa neter

Sauu-k su emment en pa neter

A tuanu ma qeti pa haru

Give thyself to ntr

Keep thou thyself daily for ntr

And let tomorrow be as today

Adorations to Sekhmet

Behold, I smell the earth before the mighty one.

Behold how I have kept the vigil in the shrine of Sekhmet. Behold, I am the child, the child of Sekhmet, the lady of the east. I am with her.

I am one with her.

I am Sekhmet and the flames of all those who praise her.

I am the hand of the powerful goddess, wearer of the solar disc.

I am the twice beautiful one, more splendid than yesterday. I am she who goes forth with Ra.

I am she.

My hair is the hair of Sekhmet, the golden one.

My eyes are the eyes of the lioness.

My ears are the ears of the goddess.

My nose is the nose of she who can sniff out all evil.

My teeth are the fangs, which can devour the darkness.

My neck is the neck of the divine goddess.

My hands are the hands with long claws.

My forearms are the forearms of the mighty one.

My backbone is golden and it shines with splendour.

My chest is the chest of the mighty one of terror.

My belly and back are the belly and back of Sekhmet.

My buttocks are strong, as the goddess.

My hips and legs are the hips and legs of the goddess.

My feet are the clawed feet of the lion goddess.

There is no part of me that is not of the goddess.

I am Sekhmet who cometh forth in the dawn.

I am the power of Ra by day.

I shall not be dragged back by my arms and none shall lay violent hands upon me, lest I destroy them utterly.

Neither man nor god shall hurt me, nor shall the living, or shall the holy dead detain me.

Nor shall the demons destroy me in battle, or I am Sekhmet and I shall eat off their faces.

I am she who cometh forth.

I am yesterday and I am the seer of millions of years.

J am the power of the divine judge.

I dwell in the east.

I am the lady of eternity, the unveiled one.

My name is created to defy all evil. I am the flame that shineth in the sanctuary. I am SEKHMET

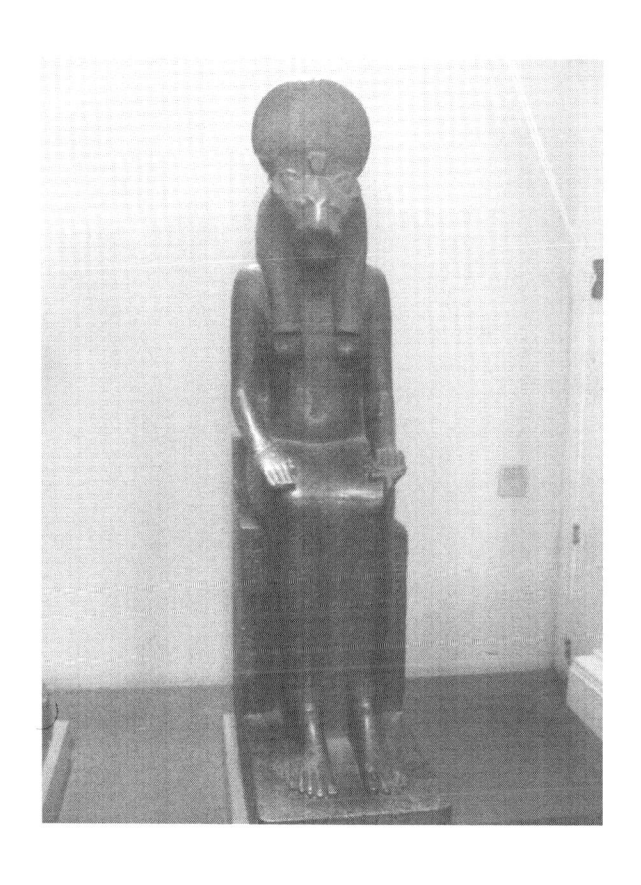

The Litany of Ra

The 75 Praises of Ra

1. Praise be unto thee, O RA, exalted Power, lord of the hidden Circles, producer of beings with forms. Thou reposest in secret habitation and performest thy creative works as the god TAMT.

2. Praise be unto thee, O RA. exalted Power, Creator, Thou spreadest out thy wings, thou restest in the TUAT (i.e. Other World or Underworld), thou givest form to the things which come forth from thy divine members.

3. Praise be unto thee, O RA, exalted Power, TA-TENEN, the begetter of the gods {of his Company]. Thou guardest what is in them, thou performest thy acts of creation as Governor of thy Circle.

4. Praise be unto thee, O RA, exalted Power, who lookest on the earth and brightenest AMENTET (the West, the Underworld). Thou art he whose attributes are his own creations; thou performest thy acts of creation in thy Great Disk.

5. Praise be unto thee, O RA, exalted Power, thou Word-soul who resteth on his high place. Thou strengthenest thy hidden AAKHIU, and they have their forms from thee.

6. Praise be unto thee, O R.A. exalted Power, mighty one, bold of face, who dost knit together thine own body. Thou dost gather together the gods of thy company when thou goest into thy Hidden Circle.

7. Praise be unto thee, O RA, exalted Power. Thou callest to thine Eye, thou speakest to thy head, thou givest breath to the souls in their places; they receive it and have their forms in him (Le. thee).

8. Praise be unto thee, O RA, exalted Power, the destroyer of thine enemies; thou dost decree destruction for the dead

9. Praise be unto thee, O RA, exalted Power. Thou sendest light, unto thy Circle, thou makest darkness to be in thy Circle, and coverest those who are therein [therewith].

10. Praise be unto thee, O RA, exalted Power, the illuminer of bodies in the horizon; thou enterest thy Circle.

11. Praise be unto thee, O RA, exalted Power, supporter of the Circles of AMENTET; thou art the body of the god TEMU

12. Praise be unto thee, O RA, exalted Power, the hidden supporter of ANPU; thou art the body of KHEPRJ

13. Praise be unto thee, O RA, exalted Power, whose existence is longer than that of her whose forms are hidden. Truly thou art the bodies of SHU.

14. Praise be unto thee, O R.A. exalted Power, the leader of RA to his members. Truly thou an the bodies of TEFNUT

15. Praise be unto thee, O RA, exalted Power, who dost make abundant the things of RA in their seasons; truly thou art GEBS

16. Praise be unto thee, O RA, exalted Power, thou mighty one, who keepest count of the things which are in him (i.e. thee). Truly thou an the bodies of NUT

17. Praise be unto thee, O RA, exalted Power, thou lord who advances! truly thou art Isis.

18. Praise be unto thee, O RA , exalted Power, whose head shineth more than what is in front of him ; truly thou art the bodies of NEPHTHYS

19. Praise be unto thee, O RA. exalted Power, who art united in thy members, One, who collectest all seed; truly thou art the bodies of HORUS.

20. Praise be unto thee, O RA, exalted Power, thou shining one, who dost send forth light upon the waters of heaven. Truly thou art the bodies of NU (NUNU)

21. Praise be unto thee, O RA, exalted Power, the avenger of NU, who comest forth from what is in him. Truly thou art the bodies of the god REMI

22. Praise be unto thee, O RA, exalted Power. Thou art the two Uraei (Cobras) who bear their two feathers (on their heads). Truly thou art the bodies of the Two HUAITI gods

23. Praise be unto thee, O RA, exalted Power. Thou goest in and earnest out, thou comest out and goest in to thy hidden Circle. Truly thou art the bodies of AATU.

24. Praise be unto thee, O RA, exalted Power, the Soul who departeth at his appointed time. Truly thou art the bodies of NETHERT .

25. Praise be unto thee, O RA, exalted Power, who standeth up, the Soul One, who avengeth his children. Truly thou art the bodies of NETUTI.

26. Praise be unto thee, O RA, exalted Power. Thou raisest thy head, and makest thy brow strong, thou Ram, strengthener of creatures.

27. Praise be unto thee, O RA, exalted Power, thou light of SHU, prince of AGERT; Truly thou art the bodies of AMENT

28. Praise be unto thee, O RA, exalted Power, the Soul that seem, the governor of AMENT. Truly thou art the bodies of the Double

29. Praise be unto thee, O RA, exalted Power. Thou art the Soul that mourneth and the god that weepeth. Truly thou art the bodies of AAKEBI.

30. Praise be unto thee, O RA, exalted Power. Thou makest thy band to pass, and praisest thine Eye. Truly thou art the bodies of the god whose limbs are hidden

31. Praise be unto thee, a RA, exalted Power. Thou art the Exalted Soul in SHETATl Truly thou art KHENTI

32. Praise be unto thee, O RA, exalted Power, of manifold forms in the Holy House. Truly thou art the bodies of the god KHEPRER

33. Praise be unto thee, O RA, exalted Power. Thou placest thine enemies in their strong fetters. Truly thou art the bodies of MATI

34. Praise be unto thee, O RA, exalted Power. Thou gives light in the hidden place. Truly thou art the bodies of the god of generation

35. Praise be unto thee, 0 RA, exalted Power, vivifier of bodies, making throats to inhale breath. Truly thou art the bodies of TE-BATI

36. Praise be unto thee, a RA, exalted Power, assembler of bodies in the TUAT, and they acquire living forms. Thou destroyest foul humours. Truly thou art the bodies of SERQI [the Scorpion god]

37. Praise be unto thee, 0 RA, exalted Power, Hidden-face SESHEM NETHERT. Truly thou art the bodies of SHAI

38. Praise be unto thee, a RA, exalted Power, lord of might, embracer of the TUAT. Truly thou art the bodies of SEKHEN-BA

39. Praise be unto thee, a RA, exalted Power, hiding thy body in what is in thee. Truly thou art the bodies of AMEN-KHAT

40. Praise be unto thee, a RA, exalted Power, stronger of heart than thy followers, sender of fire into the house of destruction. Truly thou art the bodies of REKHI

41. Praise be unto thee, 0 RA, exalted Power. Thou sendest forth destruction, and makest beings to live by thy creations in the TUAT. Truly thou art the bodies of TUATI

42. Praise be unto thee, 0 RA, exalted Power, BUA-TEP, governor of his Eye, the sender forth of light into the hidden place. Truly thou art the bodies of SHEPI.

43. Praise be unto thee, 0 RA, exalted Power, TEMT-HATU. stablisher of AMI-TA Truly thou art the bodies of TEMT-HATU

44. Praise be unto thee, 0 RA, exalted Power, creator of hidden things, generator of bodies. Truly thou art the bodies of SESHT AI

45. Praise be unto thee, O RA, exalted Power, providing those who are in the TUAT with their necessaries in the hidden Circles. Truly thou art the bodies of APER-TA

46. Praise be unto thee, O RA, exalted Power. Thy limbs rejoice when they see thy body, o UASH-BA thou enterest thy body. Truly thou art the bodies of HAI

47. Praise be unto thee, O RA, exalted Power. Thou art the Aged One of the pupil of the UDJAT, BAI Thou makest full thy splendours and thou art indeed the bodies of THENTI

48. Praise be unto thee. O RA, exalted Power. Thou makest straight paths in the TUAT, and openest up roads in the hidden places. Truly thou art the bodies of MAA-UATA

49. Praise be unto thee, O RA, exalted Power, thou Soul who advancest and hasteneth thy steps. Truly thou art the bodies of AKHPA

50. Praise be unto thee. O RA, exalted Power. Thou sendest out thy stars and lighteneth the darkness in the Circles of those whose forms are hidden. Truly thou art the bodies of HEDJIU

51. Praise be unto thee, O RA, exalted Power, maker of the Circles, maker of creatures by thine own creative force. Thou, O RA, hast created things existent and things non-existent, the dead, the gods, and the spirits. Truly thou art the Body that created KHATIU

52. Praise be unto thee. O RA, exalted Power, hidden and secret god twofold. The Souls go where thou leadest, and thy followers thou makest to enter in. Truly thou art the bodies of AMENI

53. Praise be unto thee. 0 RA, exalted Power, UBEN-AN of AMENT. The light of the lock of hair on thee .... Truly thou art the bodies of UBEN.

54. Praise be unto thee, 0 RA. exalted Power, Aged One of forms who goest through the TUAT, to whom the Souls in their Circles ascribe praises. Truly thou art the bodies of THEN-ARU

55. Praise be unto thee, 0 RA, exalted Power. When thou unitest thyself to the Beautiful AMENT the gods of the TUAT rejoice at the sight of thee. Truly thou art the bodies of AAI

56. Praise be unto thee, 0 RA, exalted Power. the Great Cat, the avenger of the gods, the judge of words [and deeds], President of the Assessors, and Governor of the Holy Circle. Truly thou art the bodies of the Great Cat

57. Praise be unto thee, 0 RA, exalted Power. When thou fillest thine Eye, and speakest to the pupil thereof, the divine dead shed tears. Truly thou art the body of METU--AAKHUT-F

58. Praise be unto thee, 0 RA, exalted Power. Thou art the Soul on high and thy bodies are hidden. Thou sendest forth light and seest thy hidden things. Truly thou art the bodies of HER-BA

59. Praise be unto thee. 0 RA, exalted Power, exalted of Soul, destroyer of thine enemies, sender of fire on the wicked. Truly thou art the bodies of QA-BA

60. Praise be unto thee. 0 RA, exalted Power. AUAlU, hider in purity. Thou art the master of the souls of the gods. Truly thou art the bodies of AUAIU

61. Praise be unto thee, O RA, exalted Power, Oldest One, Great One, governor of the TUAT , KHEPRI . Thou art the creator of the SEDJTI , whose bodies truly thou art.

62. Praise be unto thee. O RA. exalted Power, Mighty One of travels. Thou orderest thy goingsby MAAT, Thou art the Soul that doest good to the body. Thou art SENK-HRA (i.e. STI-HRA, Face of Light). Truly thou art his body.

63. Praise be unto thee, O RA. exalted Power. Thou pro-tectest thy body, and holdest the balance among the gods on the hidden AMA and AM-TA. Truly thou art the bodies of AMA AMTA

64. Praise be unto thee, O RA, exalted Power, Lord of the fetters of thine enemies, One. Prince of the Baboons Truly thou art the bodies of ANTETU

65. Praise be unto thee, O RA, exalted Power. Thou sendest fire into thy furnaces, and cuttest off the heads of those who are to be destroyed truly thou art the bodies of KETUITI

66. Praise be unto thee, O RA, exalted Power, god of generation, destroyer of thine offspring, One, stablisher of EGYPT by thy strength. Truly thou art the bodies of TA-THENEN

67. Praise be unto thee, O RA, exalted Power, Stablisher of the gods who watch the hours (URSHIU) on their standards, and are invisible and secret Truly thou art the bodies of the URSHIU

68. Praise be unto thee, O RA. exalted Power, thou DJENTI of heaven, Gate of the TUAT, and BESI/and his spirit bodies Truly thou art the bodies of BESI

69.Praise be unto thee; O RA, exalted Power.

69. Praise be unto thee; O RA, exalted Power. Thou art the Apes the true creative Power of divine attributes Truly thou art the bodies of the Ape-god in the TUAT.

70. Praise be unto thee, O RA, exalted Power, renewer of the earth, opener of the way for that which is therein, Soul giving names unto his limbs. Truly thou art the bodies of SMA-TA

71. Praise be unto thee, O RA, exalted Power, NEHI, burning up thine enemies. SEDJTI In burner of fetters. Truly thou art.the bodies of NEHI

72. Praise be unto thee, O RA, exalted Power, god of motion, god of Light, traveller bringing on darkness after the light. Truly thou an the bodies of SHEMTI

73. Praise be unto thee, O RA. exalted Power, lord of souls who art in the house of thine obelisk chief of the gods who are governors of their shrines. Truly thou art the bodies of NEB-BAlU, Lord of Souls.

74. Praise be unto thee, O RA, exalted Power, Sphinx-god, Obelisk-god, Raiser of his two Eyes. Truly thou art the bodies of HUAlTI.

75. Praise be unto thee, O RA, exalted Power, Lord of Light, Declarer of hidden things, Soul who boldest converse with the gods in their Circles. Truly thou art the bodies of NEB-SENKU (i.e. NEB-STI, Lord of Light)

(Translated by E A Wallis Budge and published in his "From Fetish to God in Ancient Egypt")

Testimonials

As a child, I knew I had a healing presence. I remember people, strangers even wanting to hug me. Wherever my parents took me there was someone stopping either of them to compliment or engage in conversation and turn to me. I noticed my elders wanted me around. When my older cousins who were shushed and told to stay in a child's place, for some reason I was allowed to remain there. I grew older and all kinds of people were attracted to me but they didn't know why. My parents weren't happy with a lot of my peers and the element in which I moved through but Compton was what it was as far as consciousness back then. The first time I experienced reiki was in West Los Angeles when my Mama was having trouble with her neck and back. I watched the practitioner as she went over my Ma's body with her hands and my Ma did say she felt the "heat". I remember it being quiet, little sun shining in and plants in the room. No speaking only the session.

From there I practiced it from a distance, sending heat or healing energy to people. I would visualize traveling through a persons body and healing them. I went on growing, experiencing life, having my Children and I found many spiritual focuses and then Nia Yaa. Nia Yaa, I watched her. I followed and read her posts and when I was sick she made me well. She made me well ridding an infection that the hospital, that's right I meant horsepital only cured. She healed my situation. I studied her posture, and her tone. I remembered the reiki session I witnessed when I was younger and was like, "wow, this is Our Science!" I immediately went into summoning the resources to afford the classes and next thing I was in a seat looking at and hearing Yaa teaching me and my other Sistars. I feel now like it was just a matter of time and that the ANKHestors wanted me with her to learn correctly.

I did and am. In my opinion, RA Sekhi is the most powerful practice anyone walking the planet could ever be realized in or obtain. My first healing session was with me.

My second, my Ma. Just last night I received my first client. Pinched nerve, chronic pain, bulging disc, depression and he said he was, "just tired". Nia Yaa taught me how to protect myself and with this situation I will need to protect myself! She taught me how to use my healing tools, colors, images, vibrations and most importantly how to stay clear and at a high vibratory status 'consistently'. And when I'm low how to charge me up! The most important thing she said to me and to each and everyone in Our Group was that, "my line is open". I give complete thanks and gratitude to Mama Yaa for staying encouraged, embracing the power of SEKHMET, her creativity and developing this program in which to heal self and others. Our formula is: clear vessel x energy = healing. Love.
~Senet Nova Kafele

To my sister please share my remarkable exsperience. My family and i drove to Philly from Fl. for level 1 and 2 kemetic reiki. The exsperience has left a profound affect on my life. Spiritually sister Nia has brought the connection that is needed for our community to effectively heal ourselves and release ways of life that have not worked. I was blessed to have several visions that sister Nia were in. To the natural eye she has been blessed by The One Most High to teal some of best soil for cultivating our now. I will never be the same and my ancestors are proud indeed. Knowing what i learned id take the same trip because it was more than worth it.

Erika Williams, Florida

The residual effects of the Maafa has caused many indigenous healing traditions to apparently be lost. Some healing traditions of antiquity survived only as dormant memories encoded in indigenous DNA. Give thanks these ancient African memories are RA-awakened in sister Kajara Nia Yaa. Ra Sekhi is the reawakening of one of the oldest healing systems humanity has brought forth. Moreover, Ra Sekhi codifies and articulates what many Afrikan wholistic practitioners tend to do intuitively. It reveals how working with spirit guides and ancestors are necessary natural aspects of a wholistic healing. It explains why wellness providers must live a principled life that embodies the wellness being imparted to others. Most importantly, Ra Sekhi outlines that principled life and inspires one to live it. It is an empowering system for Afrikan wholistic wellness providers regardless of specialty – nutrition, massage, reflex therapy, acupressure, reiki, etc. Give thanks Almighty RA for reawakening the Sekmet Lioness in the one Nia Yaa, empowering her to reestablish Maat within ourselves , family, and community. RA STAR FOR I

Ras Ben

Author of Rocks of Ages

Ra Sekhi Oath

I release all ties, bonds, and vows that are no longer serving my highest good.

I release all negative thoughts, words and actions that do not serve my highest good.

I commit to healing myself and others.

I commit to study, practice, and share the tools and techniques of Ra Sekhi Arts Temple.

I commit to doing all I can to restore MAAT on this planet, by starting with myself.

I commit to doing all I can to be a beacon of light and inspiration for my family and community.

I commit to think, speak and act in alignment with MAAT always and in all ways.

From this day forward, by
THE POWERS OF THE UNIVERSE
ASHE AMEN RA MAAT

Contact our certified teachers for level 1 & 2 classes, healing sessions, crystal therapy, ear candling and aura cleansing.

Atlanta GA:
Sat-Ra Sobukwe-SoDaye'
Website: www.khepraspa.com
Email: kheprahealingspa@gmail.com

Wash DC :
Qamarah Muhammad El-Shamesh
www.qamarahmoon.wix.com/qamarahs-healing-hands
Email: qamarahmoon@gmail.com

Toronto CA:
Ethereal Chanie-Margareta Sat En Hetet
Email: etherealchanie@gmail.com

Charlotte NC
Aura Agape
www.herbnspicewellness.com
Email: aurasendinluv@gmail.com

Birmingham AL
Sanovia Muhammad
Email: sanoviamu@att.net

South Bend IN
Lauren Markham
Email: LadyLo2u@yahoo.com

Oakland
Brenda Hudson
Email: Brendahudsonoo@aol.com

For Ra Sekhi healing sessions visit our Certified Practitioners

In Hartford CT:
Nefermul Mas   www.the-diamond-life.com
                     diamondlifeunlimited@gmail.com

Philly PA:
Angela Walker   hills7sea@aol.com
                     www.wallstreetphilly.com

Lonnie Davis   lonniemo@gmail.com

Wash DC:
Jazmyn Miles   jazmynmiles09@gmail.com
Maat Sekhem Akhita   ccpeeples@gmail.com

Charlotte NC:
Ifasayo   tite519@yahoo.com
Gagan Hunter   gaganjii@earthlink.net
                     www.gaganhunter.com

Long Beach CA:
Nova Kafele   Novakafele@gmail.com
                     Krstmoorproduce.spruz.com

Chicago IL:
Aya Posey   christaaya@gmail.com
Neffera Tresica Samuel   maaticembrace@yahoo.com

NY area
Robyn Mahone Lonesom   uhurabiz@earthlink.net
Tabia Beckett   yagottaloveus@gmail.com

Birmingham AL:
Demetrius Newton Jr.   Newpowrsol@bellsouth.net

Northern CA:
Tchiya Amet El Maat   amet13@tchiya.com
Cosmic Sound Healing   www.cosmic.tchiya.com

One of our goals is to create a community that will provide a loving, learning, and caring environment for ones to come and heal from dis-eases of the body, mind, and spirit.

This community will be eco-friendly and will include the use of solar energy, organic farming and other natural resources and techniques to ensure sustainability. The community will offer events, classes, retreats natural healing products and a variety of holistic healing modalities to facilitate healing throughout the community.

We intend to create a healthy environment for children, individuals, and families to come throughout the year to learn, share, heal and experience the beauty of and reconnect with Mother Earth.

For more info and to support this vision visit
www.gofundme.com/191dl0

For more information about our classes and events visit

www.rasekhihealing.com

Visit our sister sites as well

www.youtube.com/rasekhiartstemple

www.facebook.com/rasekhiartstemple

www.niadesigns.etsy.com

www.itsnatural.weebly.com

Ra Sekhi Arts Temple

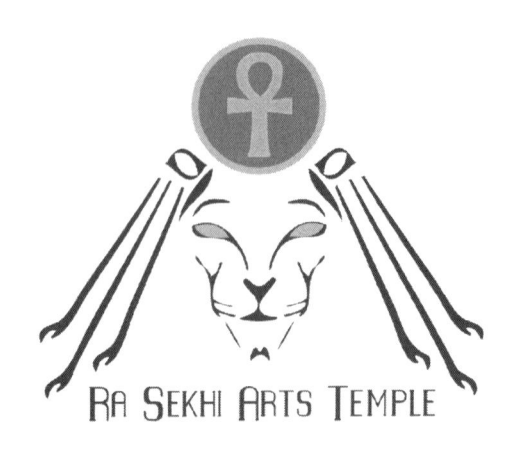

Disclaimer

RA Sekhi Arts Temple of Healing will not diagnose or attempt to cure any diseases.

Participation with RSATH is voluntary and RSATH does not accept responsibility for the management of one's health care.

RSATH does not give a medical diagnosis, prognosis or substitute for medication or medical advice.

If you are under medical supervision, you should continue under the care of my physician and not discontinue any medications without the advice of my doctor.

I have read the above and agree to abide by the conditions.

Made in the USA
San Bernardino, CA
12 February 2014